AF443473

Neck Injury

The Use of X-Rays, CTs, and MRIs to Study Crash-Related Injury Mechanisms

Jeffrey A. Pike

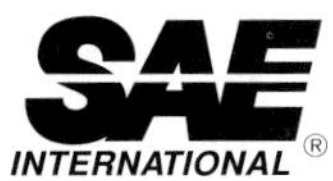

Society of Automotive Engineers, Inc.
Warrendale, Pa.

Library of Congress Cataloging-in-Publication Data

Pike, Jeffrey A.
    Neck injury : the use of x-rays, CTs, and MRIs to study
crash-related injury mechanisms / Jeffrey A. Pike.
      p. cm.
    Includes bibliographical references and index.
    ISBN 0-7680-0905-7
    1. Neck—Wounds and injuries. 2. Crash injuries.
    3. Whiplash injuries. 4. Neck—Imaging. I. Title.

RD533.5 P55 2002
617.5'3044—dc21

                                    2002021704

To

Debra

Contributors

Ronald S. Adler
Professor, Department of Radiology, Weil School of Medicine,
Cornell University
and
Attending Radiologist, Hospital for Special Surgery

Jeffrey S. Augenstein
Professor of Surgery, Division of Trauma and Surgical Critical Care
and
Director, William Lehman Injury Research Center, University of Miami
School of Medicine

Mary Ann Gregor
Senior Research Associate, University of Michigan Medical School
and
Administrative Director, University of Michigan Injury Research Center

Tristram Horton
Clinical Research Associate, William Lehman Injury Research Center
University of Miami School of Medicine

Donald F. Huelke
Professor Emeritus, Department of Anatomy, University of Michigan
Medical School
and
Senior Research Scientist Emeritus, University of Michigan
Transportation Research Institute

Ronald F. Maio
Associate Professor, Department of Emergency Medicine,
University of Michigan Medical School
and
Director, University of Michigan Injury Research Center

Jeffrey A. Pike
Senior Technical Specialist, Environmental & Safety Engineering,
Ford Motor Company
and
Adjunct Professor, Biomedical Engineering,
Wayne State University

Frank A. Pintar
Professor, Department of Neurosurgery, Medical College of Wisconsin
and
Director, Neuroscience Research Laboratories, VA Medical Center,
Milwaukee, Wisconsin

Narayan Yoganandan
Professor and Chairman, Biomedical Engineering,
Medical College of Wisconsin
and
VA Medical Center, Milwaukee, Wisconsin

Contents

Acknowledgments

Special thanks to Rick Ruth and Brian Geraghty.

Much of the material in this book has been adapted from lectures that I have given at universities; from presentations that I have made at various technical conferences and at various government and industry forums; and from lectures that I have given through the SAE Seminar Program. The attendees at these events provided much useful feedback and helped me to identify the information that would be most useful to include in this volume.

One of the most rewarding aspects of writing this book has been interacting with the very talented people mentioned below. Although very busy, they were all quite generous with their time and expertise. They taught me a great deal, not only about the subject matter, but also about graciously helping others.

The co-authors:

> Ronald S. Adler PhD MD, Jeffrey S. Augenstein MD PhD, Mary Ann Gregor MHSA, Tristram Horton BS MD IIb, Donald F. Huelke PhD, Ronald F. Maio DO, Frank A. Pintar PhD, and Narayan Yoganandan PhD.

The reviewers:

> O. Petter Eldevik MD, Mark Falahee MD, Barry Gross MD, Julius Huebner MD, Guy Nusholtz PhD, and James Szocik MD.

The following people provided various figures, radiological images, and/or case studies. The figures, of course, helped to clarify the various concepts. A great deal of effort was expended in obtaining films that were easy to read and that readily illustrated the points being made. And finally, the case studies helped to tie together the injury, radiological, and vehicle aspects of crash injury:

Ronald S. Adler PhD MD, Jeffrey S. Augenstein MD PhD, John Cavanaugh MD, Mary Ann Gregor MHSA, Tristram Horton BS MD IIb, Donald F. Huelke PhD, Ronald F. Maio DO, Frank A. Pintar PhD, Harry Smith PhD MD, and Narayan Yoganandan PhD.

Last but not least, my thanks to Martha Swiss and the Publications crew at SAE. SAE's helpfulness and professionalism in the past helped me to decide to write this second book (first book was Pike 1990), and this current collaboration has made me think in terms of book "number three."

Introduction

This book is unique in that it is intended for the wide variety of professionals involved in the study of crash-related neck injury. For those with primarily a vehicle background, it provides an overview of how x-rays, CTs, and MRIs may be used as a source of information to help analyze vehicle crashes and the associated injuries. For those with primarily a clinical background, it provides insight into how injuries relate to the vehicle crash. Determining the type of motion(s) associated with a particular injury can be of considerable importance for several reasons. These include: (1) helping to understand how to reduce the risk of such injuries in the future; (2) providing insight into how a particular injury should be treated; and (3) alerting the health-care provider to specific concomitant injuries that may be associated with a particular injury, but which are quite subtle and easy to overlook (especially initially).

This book draws upon various experiences that I have had during my 25+ years in automotive safety, especially lectures that I delivered at universities, technical societies, and government and industry forums. More specifically, the university lectures included those at Harvard Medical School, the University of Michigan, and Wayne State University. Government and industry forums included organizing and/or presenting at meetings of the Detroit Institute of Ophthalmology, Florida State Legislature, National Highway Traffic Safety Administration (NHTSA), White House Conferences, the SAE Government-Industry Meeting, and Arizona and Michigan Councils of Government. I have also had the opportunity to review research proposals for the U.S. Centers for Disease Control and review technical papers for the Association for the Advancement of Automotive Medicine, Society of Automotive Engineers (SAE), and National Academy of Sciences/Transportation Research Board. Last but not least, during the last 15 years, I have organized and presented at more than 50 SAE conferences and technical seminars.

This book is intended to provide an introduction to plain film radiographs ("x-rays"), computed tomograms, and magnetic resonance images such that vehicle safety professionals can use these techniques to help piece together the puzzle and provide a better understanding of the relationship between vehicle crash scenarios and occupant injury. It is intended to foster communication and collaboration in the increasingly complex and interdisciplinary fields of biomechanics, injury mechanism, injury mitigation, and injury treatment. The book is also intended to be of use to those safety professionals who interact with biomechanics or with EMS personnel, neurosurgeons, orthopaedists, radiologists, or other care providers. Although much of the text and almost all of the illustrations refer to the neck, many of the discussions regarding x-rays, CTs, and MRIs should be applicable to other body regions as well.

The text of this book is divided into three chapters: 1, Anatomy; 2, Imaging; and 3, Injuries and Injury Mechanisms. Chapter 1, Anatomy, provides an introduction to some anatomical, physiological, and biomechanical terminology and concepts relating to the body's structure, function, and physical limits. These terms and concepts are used in the other chapters. Chapter 2, Imaging, discusses imaging modalities encountered in the trauma environment, most notably plain film radiographs (x-rays), computed tomography (CT), and magnetic resonance imaging (MRI). The discussion describes the various views, how they are generated, and the type of injury and injury mechanism information each view may provide. Chapter 3, Injuries and Injury Mechanisms, provides a discussion about the types of injuries that can occur in a vehicle crash and the mechanisms thought to underlie them. Most of the technical terms are defined as they are introduced into the discussion; therefore, the book should be "readable" without a clinical or injury biomechanical background. However, the book also discusses some fairly advanced concepts and should be of interest to those with clinical and/or biomechanical backgrounds as well.

The topic coverage is not uniform throughout the text, but rather provides different levels of detail as appropriate to enable the reader to derive the maximum possible information from the available images and to help put the various images and case studies into context. This book has been written without seeking to provide an exhaustive (or exhausting) treatment of these very broad subjects, but rather to teach useful, important concepts and to point toward other sources. Like the cervical spine, the circumference of which varies along its length (presumably the thickness varies to accommodate the functional requirements at each level), the text varies, being more detailed for some topics than for others. It is hoped that the distribution selected will serve well, not only to address current interests, but to provide a useful framework in which to understand and apply future developments.

Chapter 1

Anatomy

JEFFREY A. PIKE
DONALD F. HUELKE

INTRODUCTION

This chapter briefly discusses some terminology and concepts relating to the structure and function of the human body and relating to injury. Many of these terms and concepts will be used in the remainder of the book.[1]

ANATOMY

The normal spine for an individual standing straight is not straight, but rather has three major curves (in the mid-sagittal plane), approximately corresponding to the cervical, thoracic, and lumbar regions (Figures 1.1 and 1.2). The most superior curve, referred to as the cervical curve, is convex ventrally and extends from the top of C2 (the apex of the odontoid process, or dens) (Figure 1.3) to the middle of T2. The cervical curve is not present at birth, but rather develops during the first year (Clemente 1985). When the spinal curvature is exaggerated, it may be indicative of some pathology. Three types of spinal curvature are kyphosis, lordosis, and scoliosis. Kyphosis is a spinal curvature that is concave anteriorly (e.g., a hump-type shape); lordosis refers to a curvature that is concave posteriorly (e.g., swayback); and scoliosis is a serpentine shape in the coronal plane (e.g., characterized by uneven shoulders and a prominent shoulder blade).

---

[1] It is anticipated that people with a wide variety of backgrounds will be using this book and that some of the material will be more familiar to some readers than to others. Those wishing a brief review of terminology such as "distal," "proximal," "mid-sagittal," and "C2" are referred to a text such as Pike 1990.

1

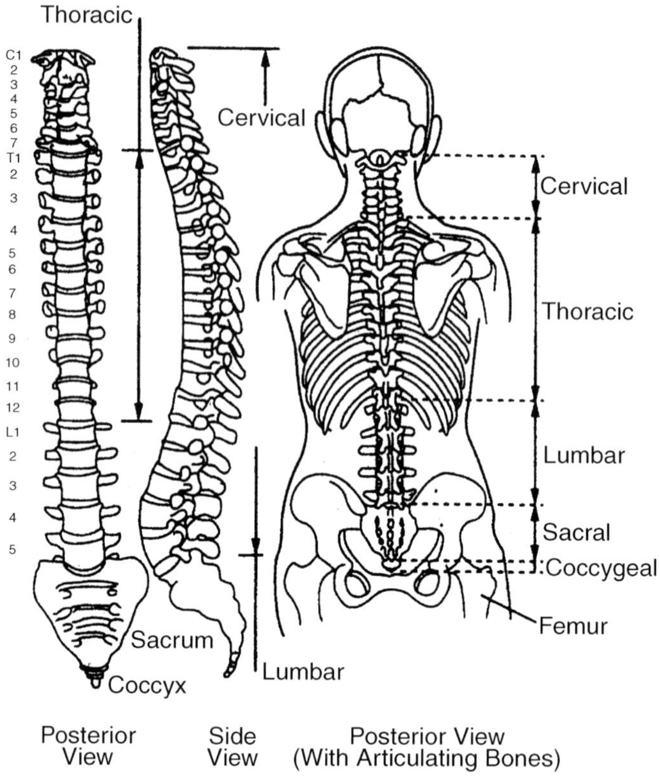

Figure 1.1   The regions of the spine.   [Reproduced with permission. Source: Pike 1990.]

The typical cervical vertebra consists of an opening in the central section of the bone, and this opening is referred to as the vertebral foramen. It is through this opening that the spinal cord passes (Figure 1.4). The cord starts at the top of the column and continues down to the lumbar region. Also, there are various ligaments (flexible, sinewy tissues that bind the vertebrae together). These ligaments connect two or more adjacent vertebrae or, in some cases, run along the length of the column. The intervertebral discs (Figures 1.2 and 1.5) are located between each vertebra in the cervical, thoracic, and lumbar regions (except for C1 and C2). Branches of the spinal cord, called nerve roots, connect the spinal cord to the face, limbs, and torso (Figure 1.6).

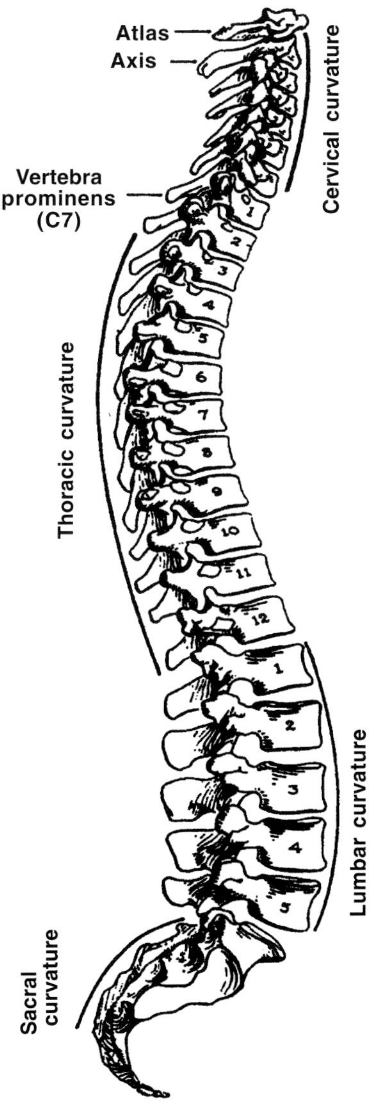

Figure 1.2 Vertebral column, lateral view. [Reproduced with permission. Source: Moore, K.E. Clinically Oriented Anatomy, *2nd Edition. Williams & Wilkins (Baltimore), 1985.]*

One of the most important characteristics of the normal spine is that adjacent vertebrae are able to move with respect to each other. When a person is standing erect, the vertebrae typically are stacked on top of each other, the front portion of each vertebra (C2 through L5) separated from the front portion of the upper and lower neighboring vertebrae (the suprajacent and subjacent vertebra, respectively) by an intervertebral disc. It is the combination of the cushion-like discs separating the vertebrae, and the sinewy ligaments tying the vertebrae together, that helps to give the vertebral column its flexibility. (The discs also help to hold the vertebrae together—each disc is firmly attached to the subjacent and suprajacent vertebrae, between which

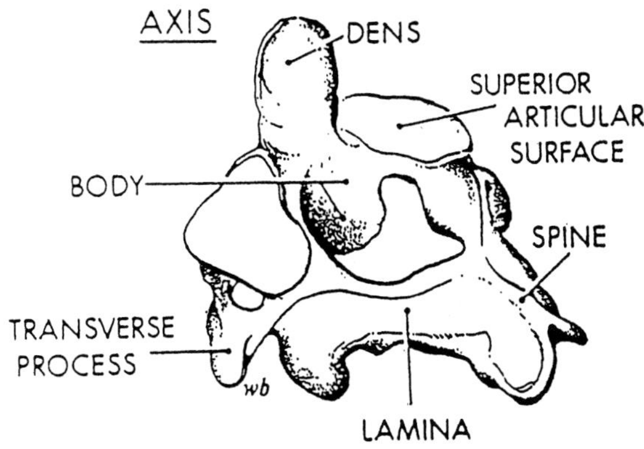

Figure 1.3 Vertebra C2 (the axis). [Reproduced with permission. Source: Huelke 1979.]

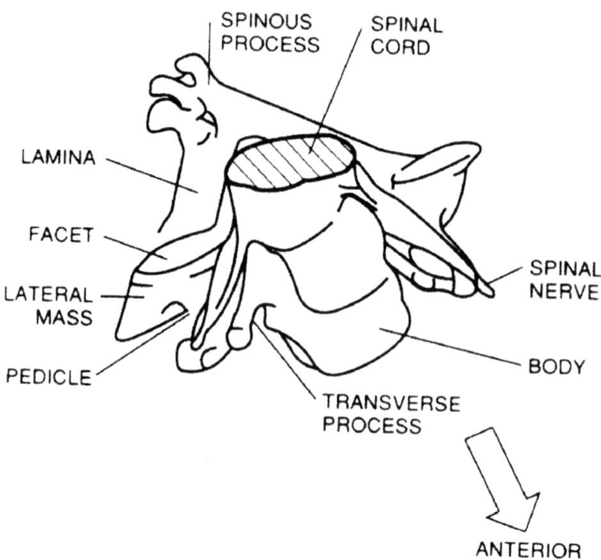

Figure 1.4   Vertebra and spinal cord.   [Reproduced with permission. Source: Pike 1990.]

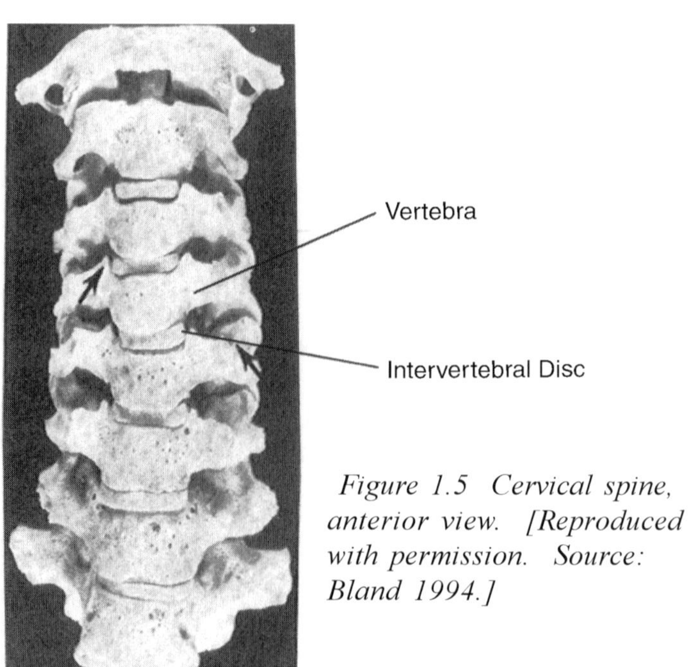

Figure 1.5 Cervical spine, anterior view. [Reproduced with permission. Source: Bland 1994.]

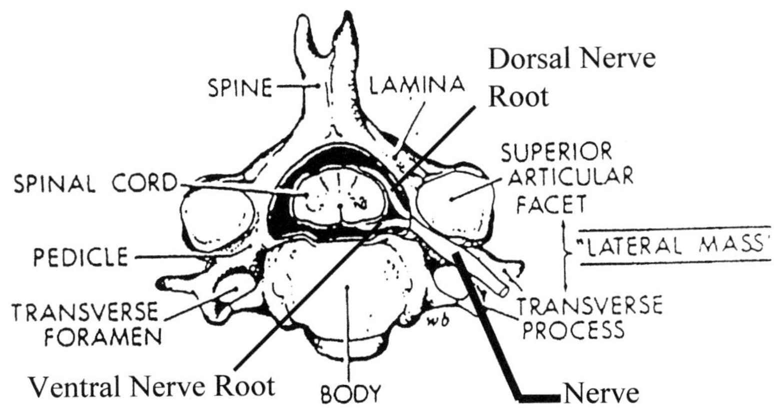

Figure 1.6 Spinal cord, spinal nerves, and nerve roots. [Reproduced with permission. Source: Huelke 1979.]

it is sandwiched.) Associated muscles provide movement and additional stability. Adjacent vertebrae articulate, in the lateral part of the vertebrae, via protrusions called articular facets. Each vertebra has a left and a right articular facet on its upper surface (the superior articular facet) (Figures 1.7 and 1.8) and a left and a right articular surface on its lower surface (the inferior articular facet) (Figure 1.8), and facets of adjacent vertebrae move against each other. For example, part of the upper surface of C5 contacts and moves against part of the lower surface of the vertebra above it, namely, C4. More specifically, the superior articular facets of vertebra C5 articulate with the inferior articular facets of vertebra C4. The facet joints are also referred to as interfacetal or zygoapophyseal joints.

As mentioned previously, the vertebrae typically have a body anteriorly and an arch posteriorly and lateral masses where the body and arch intersect, but the vertebrae tend to differ between regions and even within each region. This is especially true for the vertebrae at each end of a region, which tend, in some respects, to be transition vertebrae, between the structure and function of the two regions. Thus, the cervical region might easily be divided into an upper and lower cervical region. The upper cervical region may be thought of as providing a transition zone between the base of the skull and the remainder of the vertebral column. (The base of the skull is sometimes conceptually included as part of the vertebral column and, in keeping with this, may be referred to as "C0" [C-Zero].) The upper cervical column consists of the

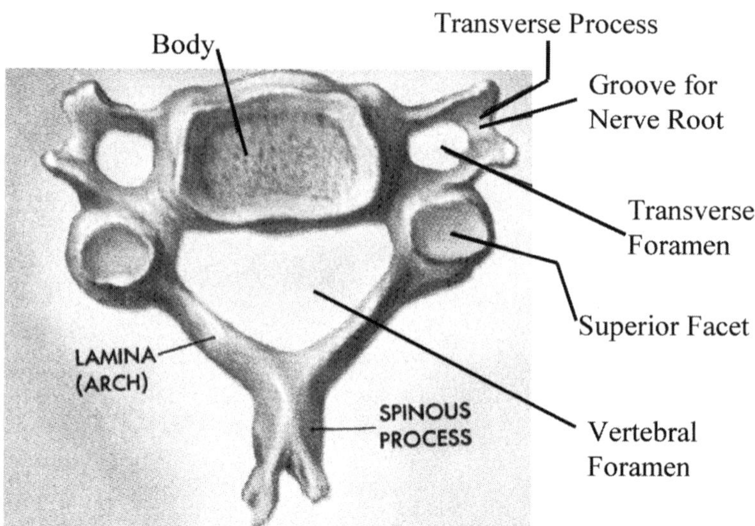

Figure 1.7 Cervical vertebra C4, body and arch. [Copyright 1972. ICON Learning Systems, LLC, a subsidiary of MediMedia USA Inc. Reprinted with permission from ICON Learning Systems, LLC, illustrated by Frank H. Netter, MD. All rights reserved.]

first two cervical vertebrae, C1 and C2. These vertebrae have very specialized functions and have structures that are quite distinct from those of the remaining cervical vertebrae (and from each other). The cervical spine may also be considered to be divided into three regions: the upper cervical column, as before, C1 and C2, providing the transition between skull and cervical vertebral column; and the remainder divided into a mid-cervical region (C3–C5) and a lower cervical region (C6 and C7). The lower cervical region provides a transition between the cervical and thoracic spine.

Structure of C1

The first cervical vertebra, the atlas, articulates with the lower surface of the skull (the occipital condyles) and supports the weight of the head. As one might expect, the superior surface of each of its articular masses (pillars) is shaped and oriented to facilitate this function (Figures 1.9 and 1.10).

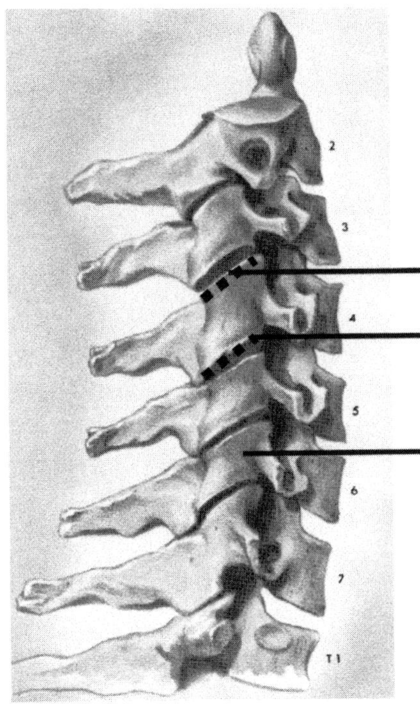

Figure 1.8 Articular surfaces. [Copyright 1972. ICON Learning Systems, LLC, a subsidiary of MediMedia USA Inc. Reprinted with permission from ICON Learning Systems, LLC, illustrated by Frank H. Netter, MD. All rights reserved.]

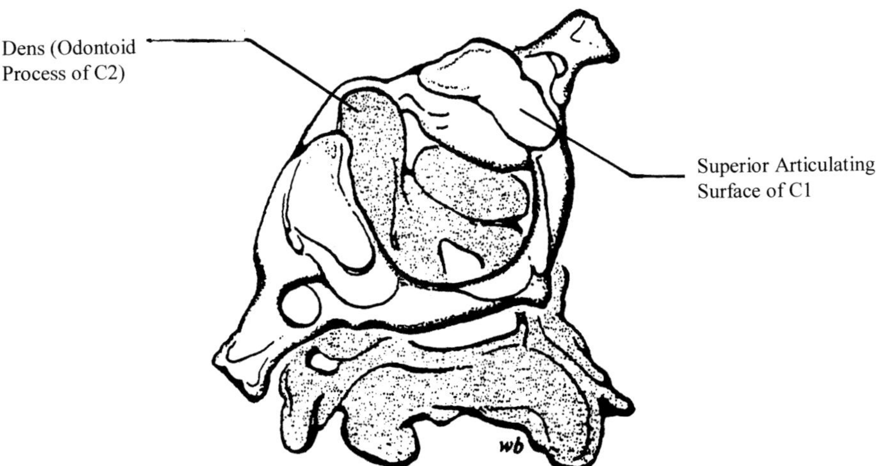

Figure 1.9 Vertebra C1 (the atlas) and vertebra C2 (the axis). [Reproduced with permission. Source: Huelke 1979.]

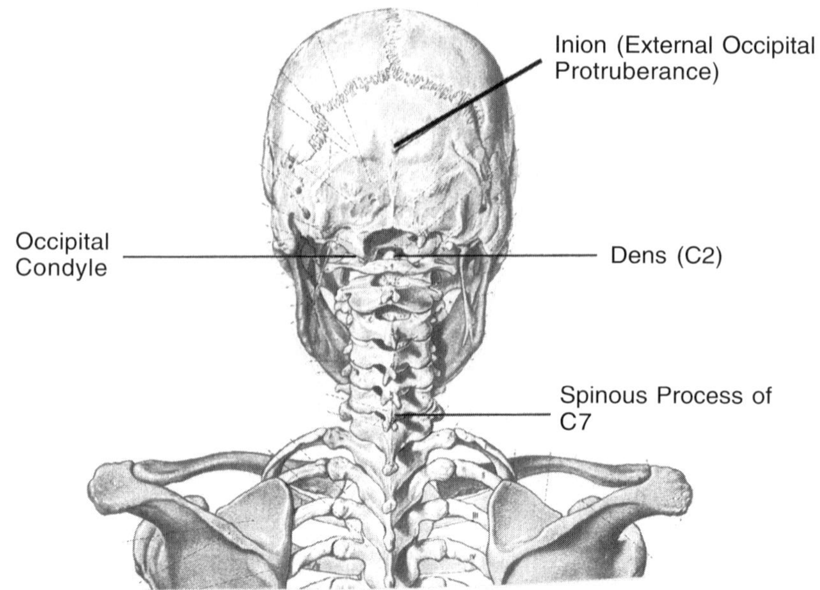

Figure 1.10   Skull and cervical spine—posterior view.   [Reproduced with permission.   Source: Pernkopf 1963.]

Structure of C2

The second cervical vertebra, the axis, is shaped quite differently from all the other cervical vertebrae. Perhaps its most distinguishing feature is a vertical structure, the odontoid process or dens (Figure 1.3), which provides a post or axis about which the atlas can rotate (Figures 1.5 and 1.9). The superior-most region of the dens is its apex. The dens passes through an expanded opening (the vertebral foramen) in the center of C1, which accommodates both the dens and the spinal cord. When the neck does rotate (a "no" gesture), most of the rotation takes place between the atlas and axis. Similar to the typical vertebra, the axis has a superior and inferior articular process on both the right and left sides.

The lower cervical spine, that is, C3 through C7, is also involved with flexion and extension movements. The lower cervical vertebrae are also involved in lateral bending, that is, moving the head from side to side and to a very limited extent, axial rotation (a "no" gesture).

Structure of C3–C7

The structure of the vertebrae of the lower cervical spine may be divided into a vertebral body anteriorly and a vertebral arch posteriorly (Figure 1.7). The vertebral body, sometimes referred to as the centrum, is nearly oval in shape and is the largest part of the vertebra. The superior and inferior surfaces of the body have a rough central area with a smooth and slightly elevated rim (Figure 1.7). (The intervertebral discs attach to the upper and lower surfaces of the body.) The vertebral arch consists of two pedicles (very short structures projecting posteriorly and slightly laterally from the vertebral body) (Figures 1.7 and 1.8). Projecting laterally from each pedicle is an articular mass, and projecting postero-medially from each lateral mass is a thin, rectangular lamina. The laminae join posteriorly, and the spinous process projects posteriorly from this junction (Figure 1.7).

The typical vertebra also has seven processes (projections used for muscle attachment) arising from the vertebral arch: four articular (from the articular facets discussed previously), two transverse, and one spinous (Figure 1.7). Two projections, the anterior and posterior transverse tubercles, extend posterolaterally from the transverse process (Figure 1.7). The transverse process is also characterized by an opening, the transverse foramen (Figure 1.7), through which the vertebral arteries are routed (except at C7, where the foramen frequently contains the accessory vertebral vein).

As mentioned previously, the rearward projection from the arch, in the midsagittal plane, is called the spinous process. It is the spinous process and the soft tissue covering it that are being felt when the backbone is manually palpated. Cervical vertebrae C3 through C7 are relatively similar in shape. C3 through C6 have spinous processes that are short and frequently fork posteriorly to form a bifid spinal process (Figure 1.7), whereas the process of C7 provides the greatest posterior projection. It is therefore the most prominent and has earned the name "vertebra promenens" for C7 (Figures 1.11 and 1.8).

There are four primary joints where adjacent vertebrae of the lower cervical spine articulate: one each on the right and left sides of the intervertebral disc and one between each of the two articular pillars. The lateral region of the raised lip at the periphery of the superior surface of the vertebral body is named the uncinate process. The articulation of the uncinate process with the edge of the inferior surface of the suprajacent vertebra is called the uncovertebral joint (also called the joint of Luschka)[2] (Figure 1.12). The joint between contiguous

---

[2] Note that the terminology for this region might be changing to reflect the recent opinion that this structure does not satisfy the strict definition of joint (Bland 1994).

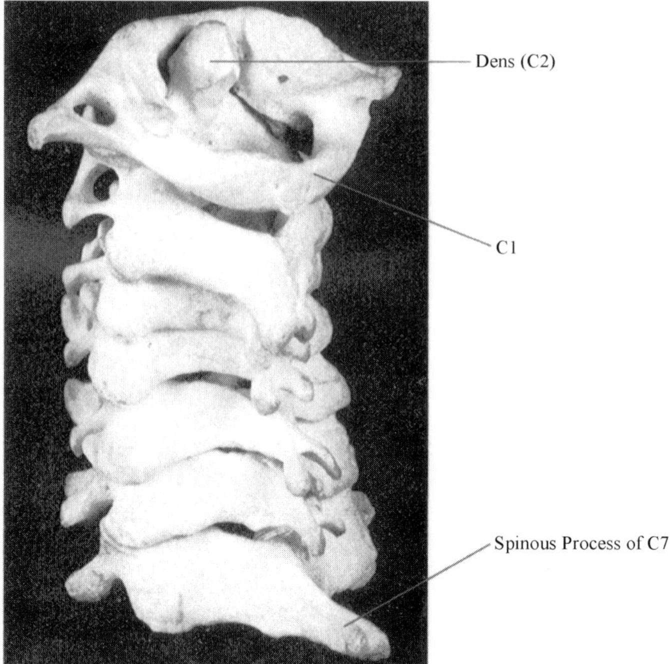

Figure 1.11 Cervical spine, posterolateral view. [Reproduced with permission. Source: Sherk, H.H. The Cervical Spine, 2nd Edition. Lippincott (Philadelphia), 1989.]

articular masses, the facet joint, is composed of the inferior surface (facet) of the superior vertebra and the superior surface (facet) of the inferior vertebra. Each vertebra has a right and a left facet (Figures 1.11 and 1.8). Thus, for each vertebra, there are a total of four facet joints (upper right, upper left, lower right, and lower left). Each of these four joints has a joint capsule, a covering of fibrous tissue. The cervical facet capsules tend to have more slack than the capsules in the lower spinal regions and therefore tend not to be as restrictive of relative motion between the articulating facets.

In addition to the joint capsules, the cervical vertebrae are tied together by a number of ligamentous structures—the vertebral bodies by the intervertebral discs, the anterior longitudinal ligament, and the posterior longitudinal ligament; the lamina by the ligamenta flava; the spinous processes by the interspinous ligament and the ligamentum nuchae (cervical extension of supraspinous ligament) (Figures 1.13 and 1.14).

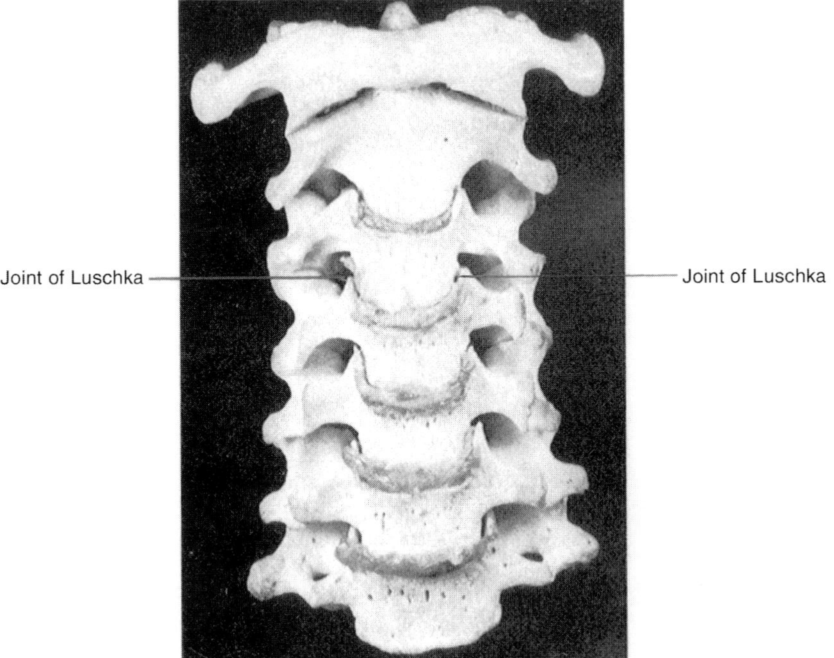

*Figure 1.12   Joints of Luschka.   [Reproduced with permission.
Source: Sherk, H.H.   The Cervical Spine, 2nd Edition.
Lippincott (Philadelphia), 1989.]*

The anterior longitudinal ligament (ALL) is attached to the anterior surface of the vertebral bodies and at the discs. The ALL is of relatively uniform width and thickens distal to the discs (i.e., is thickest midway between the discs [Figures 1.13 and 1.14]). The ALL runs the entire length of the spine (Parke 1989).

The posterior longitudinal ligament (PLL) (Figure 1.13) is widest in the upper cervical spine and narrows caudally. In addition, the PLL varies locally, being more narrow over the vertebral bodies and wider behind the vertebral discs (Parke 1989).

The ligamenta flava (LF) (Figure 1.13) attach at the lamina—the inner surface of the upper lamina and the upper margin of the lower lamina. These ligaments meet mid-sagittally and extend laterally to the articular processes, where they intertwine with the facet joint capsule (Young 1991).

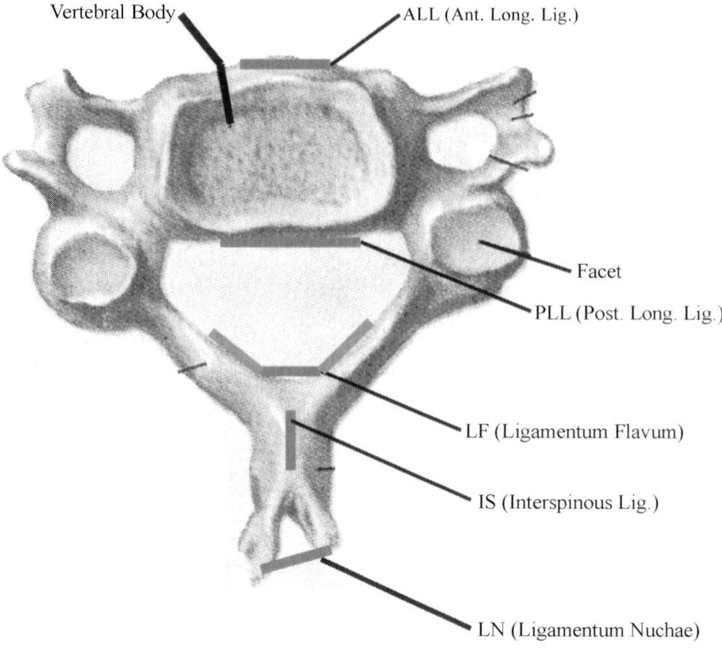

Figure 1.13 Vertebral ligaments, superior view. [Copyright 1972. ICON Learning Systems, LLC, a subsidiary of MediMedia USA Inc. Reprinted with permission from ICON Learning Systems, LLC, illustrated by Frank H. Netter, MD. All rights reserved.]

The ligamentum nuchae (LN) (Figures 1.13 and 1.14) extends from the base of the skull (more specifically, the external occipital protuberance, also called the inion) (Figure 1.10) to the spinal process of C7. Below C7, this ligament in effect continues as the supraspinous ligament (Figure 1.13).

The interspinous ligaments (IS) (Figures 1.13 and 1.14) essentially lie between the ligamenta flava and the ligamentum nuchae and extend the length of the spinous processes.

As mentioned previously, the vertebral arteries are routed through an opening in the transverse process, the transverse foramina, of C1 through C6 (Figure 1.6) and supply the spinal cord via the spinal arteries. The three spinal arteries are oriented longitudinally along the surface of the cord: the anterior spinal artery is located mid-sagittally, and the two posterior spinal arteries are symmetrically displaced from the midline (Figure 1.15).

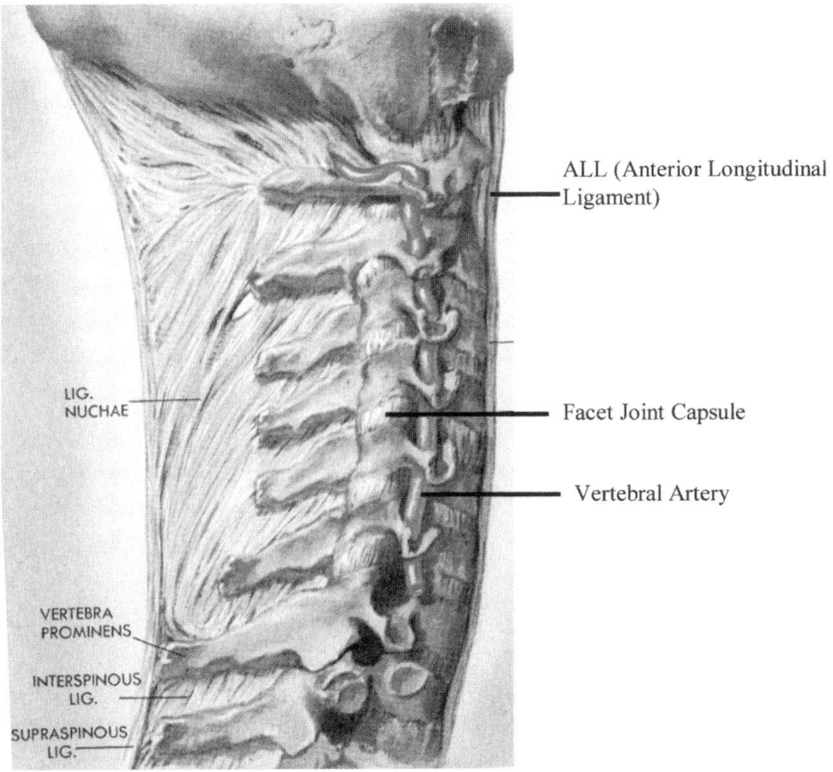

Figure 1.14 Vertebral ligaments, sagittal view. [Copyright 1972. ICON Learning Systems, LLC, a subsidiary of MediMedia USA Inc. Reprinted with permission from ICON Learning Systems, LLC, illustrated by Frank H. Netter, MD. All rights reserved.]

SPINAL INJURIES (PHYSIOLOGY, BIOMECHANICS, AND RELATED PATHOLOGY)

Most spinal injuries can be categorized as a sprain, disc disruption, vertebral fracture, or vertebral dislocation, and any one of these may or may not involve the spinal cord or spinal nerve roots. As will be discussed later, these different injury categories are by no means mutually exclusive. Indeed, injury to the various non-neural spinal structures (i.e., muscles, ligaments, discs, and

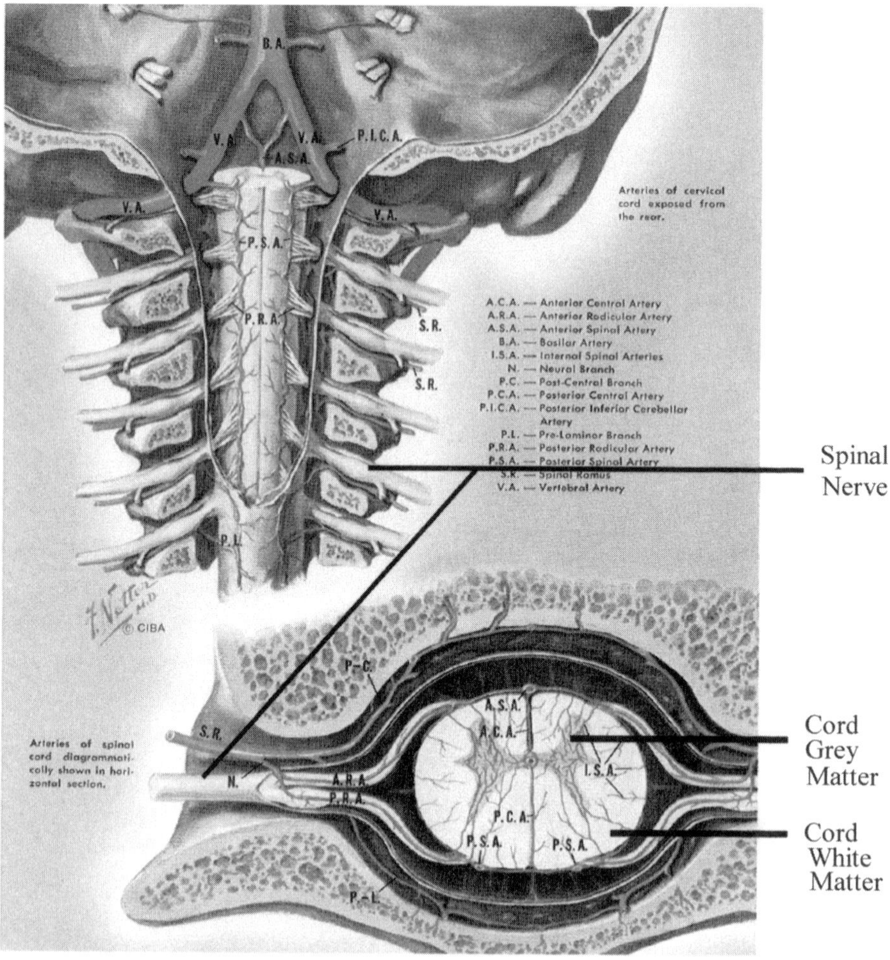

Figure 1.15 Arteries of the spinal cord. [Copyright 1972. ICON Learning Systems, LLC, a subsidiary of MediMedia USA Inc. Reprinted with permission from ICON Learning Systems, LLC, illustrated by Frank H. Netter, MD. All rights reserved.]

vertebra) generally become much more significant if they affect the neural elements—the spinal nerves and especially the spinal cord.

A sprain basically refers to the stretching of soft tissue beyond its elastic limit (that is, to such an extent that it will not return to its original shape and size, even though the stretching force is discontinued) so that it begins to tear. The soft tissue involved most often is a muscle, ligament, or facet joint capsule (that is, the fibrous structure enclosing a facet joint).

Disc disruption most frequently refers to a tearing or compression of the intervertebral disc, possibly with the extrusion of some of the contents. The fracture of a vertebra refers to an actual cracking or breaking of one of these bones.

The various injuries discussed previously often are due NOT to some unique movement, which is exclusively associated with injury, but rather are due to extremes of the various movements (and the resulting loads), which are part of normal functioning of the spine. The movements include flexion, extension, lateral flexion (lateral bending), rotation, and combinations thereof.[3]

In a vehicular crash environment, although a particular neck motion may predominate (e.g., someone may sustain what is basically a flexion-type injury), it is unlikely that the neck will undergo a single, pure motion. In fact, the spine can be injured as the result of many different complex motions. These movements may include different motions in different regions. For example, one segment of the spine may be undergoing flexion, while another segment is undergoing extension. The motion may also include a time sequence of more than one motion (e.g., a given region of the spine may first undergo flexion and then undergo extension).

As mentioned, the spinal cord, contained within the framework of the bony spine, is of ultimate concern with regard to injury. A spinal injury may involve either the spinal cord, per se, or its branches, the spinal nerve roots. When these neurological structures are damaged, loss of sensation or motor function may occur. Thus, vertebral fracture, per se, is not sufficient to cause neurological deficit. (Indeed, approximately 60% of cervical fractures have no associated neurological injury [Mahoney 1988].) Thus, a so-called broken neck (fracture of one or more cervical vertebrae), although serious in its own right, becomes much more severe if the bone is broken in such a way that the bone then injures the spinal cord (Figure 1.16).

Generally, when a vertebral fracture is such that it has the potential to cause (additional) neurological injury, the condition is referred to as being neurologically unstable or simply unstable. For the remainder of this discussion, a stable spine may be defined as a vertebral column, which during normal

---

[3] In addition to these movements, the cervical spine may be loaded externally (e.g., by an impact to the top of the head) in compression or tension, that is, a compressive or stretching force may be exerted along the length of the spine.

activity would not be expected to produce further damage to itself or to adjacent structures.[4]

Rather than direct mechanical trauma to the cord per se (e.g., impingement on the cord by displaced or fragmented vertebra or disc), neck trauma may initially injure the blood vessels supplying the cord. These types of vascular injuries may be exacerbated if there is already some spinal canal compromise due to degenerative changes (e.g., buckling of the PLL) or various diseases (e.g., bony spurs [osteophytes] associated with arthritis), which, in effect, narrow the spinal canal). (Preexisting conditions [e.g., diabetes] that limit circulatory capacity may also predispose to vascular injury).[5]

Also note that preexisting conditions might limit a person's ability to recover from trauma. For example, an older person may be more likely to succumb to a given injury than a younger, otherwise healthy individual (Pike 1989).

Cord injury may not only be indirect, but may be late (i.e., may manifest at some time subsequent to the initial physical insult). Indirect mechanisms include hypoxemia, edema, continued pressure on the cord due to mass lesion (e.g., hematoma), or shock (Mahoney 1988). Such mechanisms tend eventually to compromise the cord's blood supply and thereby produce cord ischemia (inadequate blood supply) and eventually necrosis (death of cord tissue).

---

[4] This expectation may be long term as well as short term.

[5] Various conditions, whether primarily congenital, or disease- or age-related, can predispose a person to injury. For example, atlanto-axial subluxation, a partial dislocation of the first and second cervical vertebrae, may be a complication of a variety of conditions, including rheumatoid arthritis, ankylosing spondylitis, tuberculosis, arthritis, paraspinous inflammation, or congenital anomalies of the odontoid process, such as that associated with Down's syndrome (Orrison 1989). An example of vertebral fracture in a patient with ankylosing spondylitis is provided in Figure 1.17. (Note the lack of disc space between adjacent vertebrae.) A variety of systemic diseases, which affect bones in general, can cause alterations to the cervical spine in particular. In addition to osteoporosis, these include anemias, leukemias, Hodgkin's disease, and Paget's disease (Bohlman 1986). The anemias and leukemias may reduce bone density and thereby make the bone subject to easy fracture; Hodgkin's disease may involve fracture and hence protrusion of bone and/ or tumor into the spinal canal, or there may be direct invasion of neural structures without any bony involvement; Paget's disease may initially destroy bone and then later, when bone is replaced, the resulting bone will be irregular (and susceptible to injury) (Bohlman 1986). Degenerative changes, such as osteoporosis, may also weaken the bones. Figures 1.18 and 1.19 provide a comparison of the structure of a normal and an osteoporotic vertebra. (Note that Figure 1.19 also shows other degenerative changes, namely, decrease in the disc height [disc space narrowing] and the growth of osteophytes [bony spurs].) A wide variety of conditions, e.g., coronary artery disease, gallstones, temporomandibular joint arthritis, and depression (Bland 1994) may cause referred neck pain (i.e., the neck, per se, is not injured, but the pain is perceived as originating from the neck). Such conditions, if preexisting but previously asymptomatic, may produce neck pain in response to a minor trauma that might otherwise be uneventful.

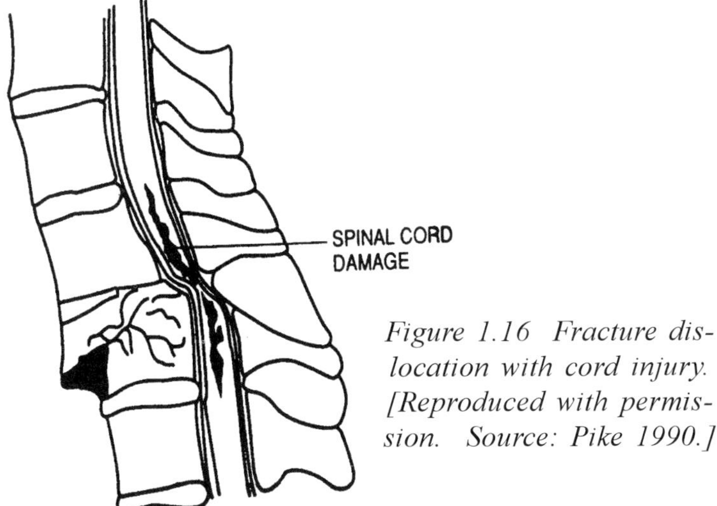

*Figure 1.16 Fracture dis-
location with cord injury.
[Reproduced with permis-
sion. Source: Pike 1990.]*

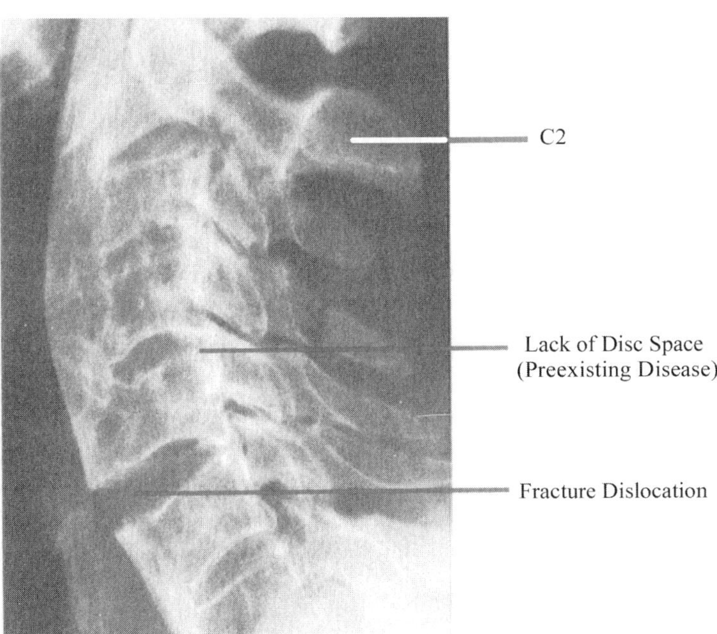

*Figure 1.17 Ankylosing spondylitis. [Reproduced with permission.
Source: Mirvis, S.E.; Young, J.W.R.* Imaging in Trauma and
Critical Care. *Williams & Wilkins (Baltimore), 1992.]*

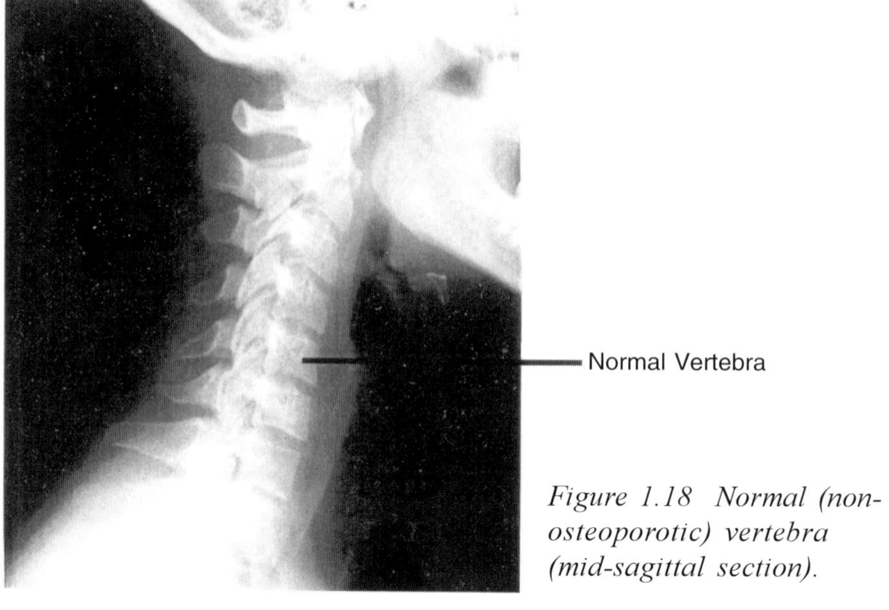

Figure 1.18 Normal (non-osteoporotic) vertebra (mid-sagittal section).

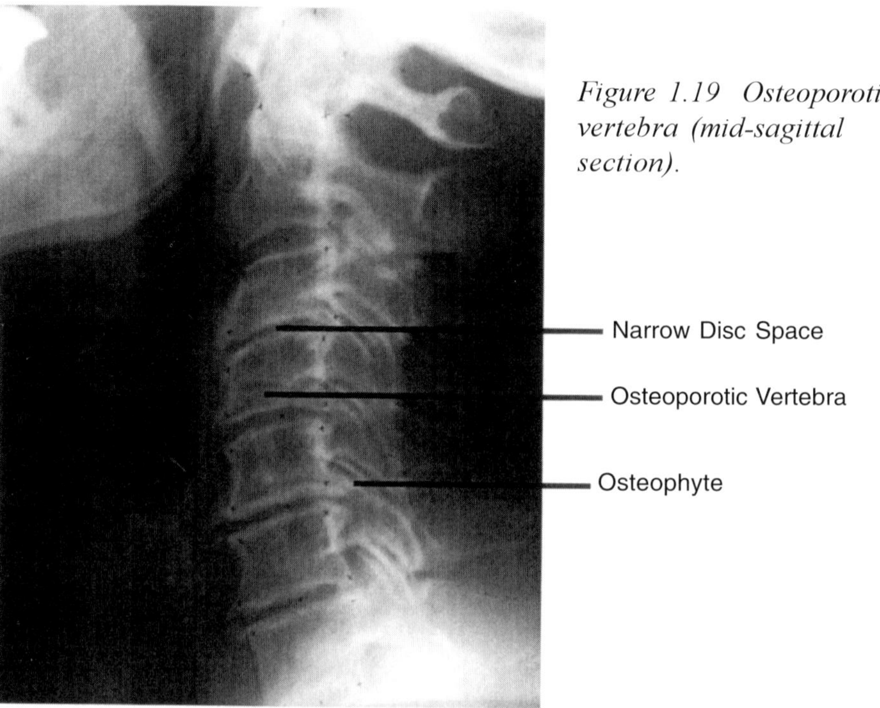

Figure 1.19 Osteoporotic vertebra (mid-sagittal section).

It is also possible for late cord injury to occur subsequent to surgery. For example, a laminectomy (removal of laminae) may be performed to relieve cord compression, and years later the weakened region (where the surgery was performed) may permit sufficient vertebral movement (e.g., dislocation) to cause neurological deficits (Bland 1994). One reason for this is that the laminectomy also removes the ligamenta flava and may damage the facet joints. Initially, other bonds (e.g., the vertebral bonding with the intervertebral disc) may be strong enough to compensate for this, but the intervertebral bond may decrease with time.

A major concern regarding a torn or ruptured disc is whether or not the content of the disc (the nucleus pulposus) is extruded rearward, to the extent that it presses on a spinal nerve (a branch of the spinal cord), or possibly even presses on the spinal cord itself (Figure 1.20). Part of the disc material may press against and possibly injure the spinal cord or spinal nerves. Depending on the extent and nature of the extrusion of this material against the neural tissue, some paralysis and loss of sensation may result.

Note that in the cervical spine, cord injury from disc protrusion is relatively unlikely. The uncinate processes act as natural barriers to posterolateral extrusion of disc material, thereby helping to prevent nerve root compression. Furthermore, the cervical nerve roots do not pass over the intervertebral discs

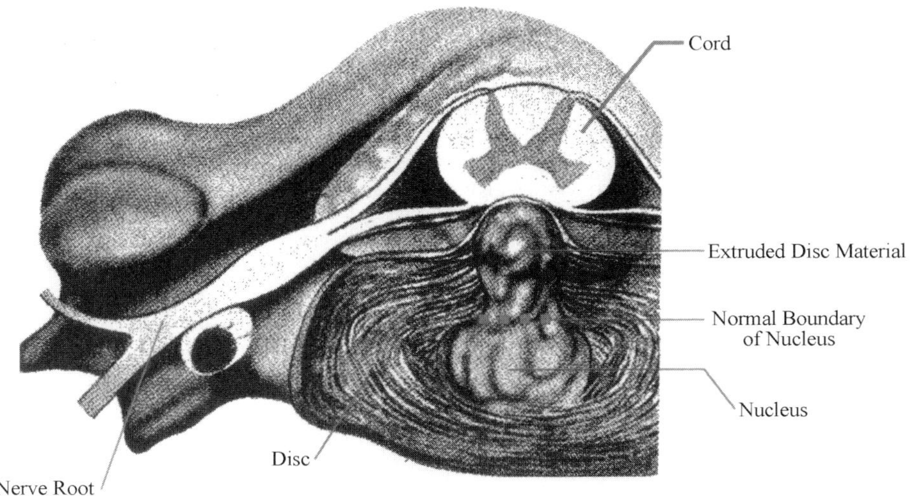

Figure 1.20 Spinal cord compression by disc. [Reproduced with permission. Source: Boden 1991.]

(in contrast to the lumbar nerve roots, which pass directly over the discs) and hence are much less prone to injury from disc protrusion (Bland 1994).

Although the spinal ligaments normally help to support the vertebral column and thereby protect the spinal cord, under certain circumstances a spinal ligament may push against the cord. This is particularly true in the elderly, in whom the ligamentum flavum is prone to buckle (Hockberger 1988). During neck extension, the ligamentum flavum may push against the cord and produce an injury, most typically to the inner diameter of the cord (Duckworth 1984). (This injury, called the central cord syndrome, is discussed later in this chapter.) Consequently, the overriding concern with regard to injuries of the discs and ligaments is essentially the same as for fractures of the vertebrae— namely, will they cause injury to the spinal cord (or one of the peripheral nerves emerging from either side of the cord)?

Two of the major functions of the spinal cord are to: (1) transmit instructions to the various muscles and organs of the body (thereby including in its functions motor activity such as walking and control [autonomic] functions such as blood pressure regulation), and (2) relay sensory information from various areas of the body to the brain, thereby enabling us to feel pressure, pain, vibration, etc. Sensory information tends to move upward (superiorly) along the spinal cord, toward the brain (cephalad), and motor information tends to move downward (inferiorly), away from the brain (caudal).

A complete disruption (transection) of the spinal cord, at any particular level, not only disrupts the functioning of the spinal cord at the site of transection, but disrupts spinal cord function, both sensory and motor, for *all parts of the spinal cord inferior to the point of injury.*

Thus, the more superior the location of a given cord injury, the more serious that injury is in terms of the extent of loss of spinal cord function (Table 1.1). Because the cervical region of the spinal cord is closest to the brain, a complete transection of the cord in this region is the most severe; it produces a loss of functioning of the sacral region, plus a loss of the functioning of the entire lumbar region, plus a loss of the entire thoracic region, plus the additional loss associated with the functioning of the affected segment of the cervical region. Thus, a spinal cord transection at the C4 level would be equivalent to the loss due to a transection at the C5 level, plus the additional loss of the functioning of the cord segment from C5 to C4.[6]

---

[6] In contrast to spinal cord injury, spinal nerve (or nerve root) (Figures 1.6, 1.21) injury does not affect the cord, nerves, or nerve roots distal to the injury site, and hence does not affect the body regions served by nerves that branch from the cord inferior to the injury site.

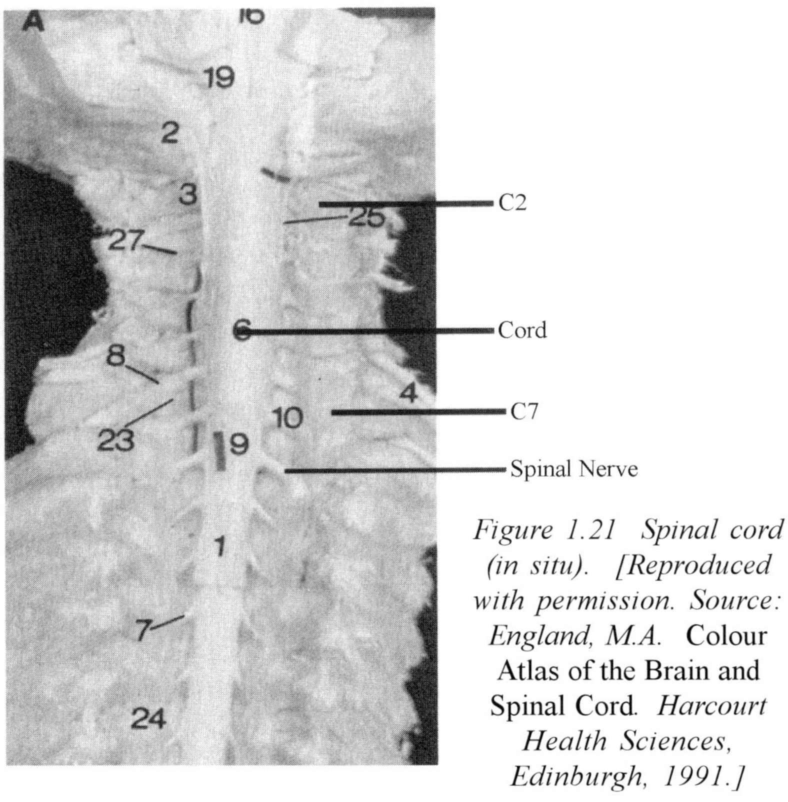

Figure 1.21 Spinal cord (in situ). [Reproduced with permission. Source: England, M.A. Colour Atlas of the Brain and Spinal Cord. *Harcourt Health Sciences, Edinburgh, 1991.]*

Table 1.1 Level of Cord Injury v. Affected Motor Function

Level of Cord Injury[7]	Typical Function Affected
QUADRIPLEGIA	
C3	Can't breathe. No motor function, all limbs.
C4	Can breathe (shallow), shrug shoulder.
C5	Can move shoulder. Some elbow movement (flexion).
C6	Can move elbow. Some wrist movement (extension).
C7	Can move wrist. Some finger movement (extension). Some hand grasp.
C8	More hand grasp. Finger flexion.
PARAPLEGIA	
T1	Upper limbs OK, lower limbs affected.

[7] Level refers to spinal nerve level, which is not identical to vertebral level—spinal nerves C1 through C7 are located near the top of the correspondingly numbered vertebrae, and the C8 nerve is located between C7 and T1.

While an embryo is developing, structures called somites each form three other structures—a sclerotome, a myotome, and a dermatome. For this discussion, perhaps the major significance of the various "tomes" is that as a result of their common embryologic origin, they remain linked in adulthood (Sadler 1985; Guyton 1987). When the embryo matures, each level of the spinal cord is associated with innervation of particular regions of the body. The region of the body's surface (cutaneous region) that sends sensory information to a given cord level is referred to as a dermatome (Figure 1.22); the muscular fibers that are innervated by the nerves from a given cord level are referred to as a myotome; and the bones and joints innervated by a given cord level are referred to as a sclerotome (Figure 1.23). (The term "angiotome" is sometimes used to refer to the blood vessels innervated by a given cord level [Byrne 1990].) The regions of the skin that incrementally would lose sensation due to a spinal cord or spinal nerve injury at the C6 level are labeled in Figure 1.22. Figure 1.23 indicates the dermatome, myotome, and sclerotome corresponding to cord level C6. Note that this agrees with the dermatomes

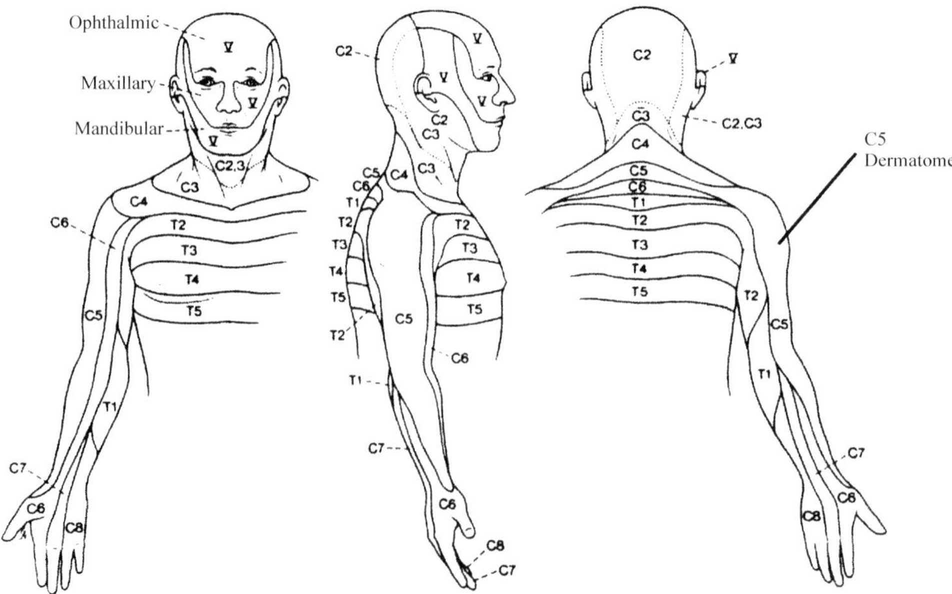

Figure 1.22 Dermatomes.   [Reproduced with permission. Source: Bland 1994.]

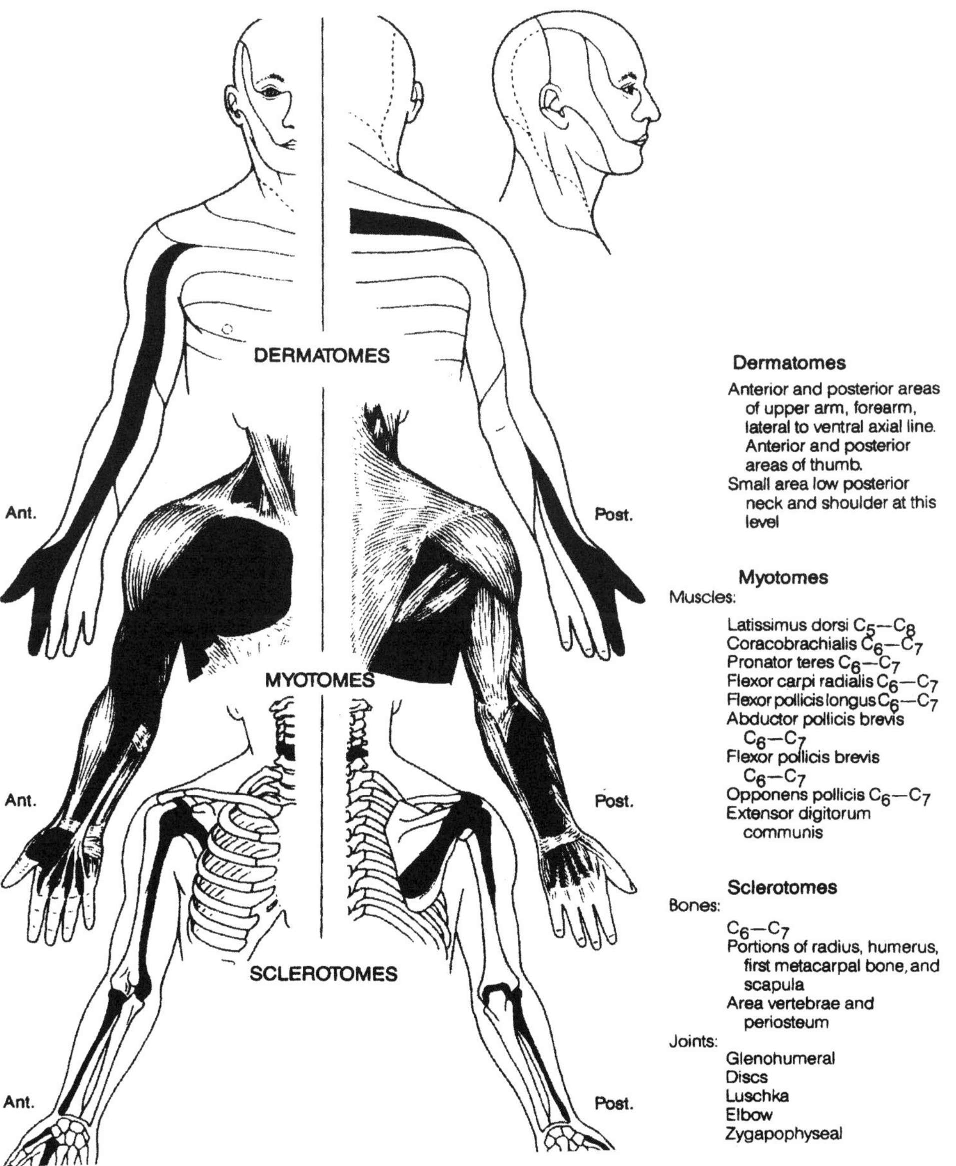

Figure 1.23 Dermatomes, myotomes, and sclerotomes.
[Reproduced with permission.   Source: Bland 1994.]

indicated in Figure 1.22 and also indicates that although the dermatomes, myotomes, and sclerotomes for a given segment are somewhat similar, they are not identical.

As has already been discussed, injury to the spinal cord or spinal nerves has far-reaching consequences with regard to loss of sensation and motion of remote regions of the body. Another consequence of the developmental linking, however, is that injury to structures, which are remote but have the same embryologic origin (and hence the same cervical nerve root innervation), may be experienced as pain in the neck region (Bland 1994). This phenomenon is sometimes described as referred pain. For example, an injury to the left trapezius muscle (in the left shoulder blade region) may be experienced as pain in the ipsilateral (left) posterolateral region of the neck (Zohn 1988).

One function of the spinal cord is to help regulate blood flow, including to itself, and thus an injury to the cord may interfere with its blood supply and thereby start a metabolic process that can lead to cord death within a few hours. Secondary injury from altered blood flow regulation is a very important aspect of cord injury, because it means that therapeutic intervention may be possible within those first few hours to minimize or eliminate the long-term deficits currently associated with that type of cord injury. New medications (e.g., CM-101) (Wamil 1998), are being explored to see if early intervention can ameliorate the outcome of cord trauma.

As a general guideline, the cervical region of the spinal cord controls the upper torso and upper extremities; the thoracic region controls the lower torso; the lumbar region controls the lower limbs and contributes to urination; and the sacral region controls defecation and urination and contributes to ambulation (walking). (Actually, the cord per se does not extend into the sacral region [in adults, it stops around L-2], but a hair-like extension of the cord, the cauda equina, extends into the upper sacral region.) Other possible consequences of cord injury include neurogenic bladder dysfunction (i.e., urinary bladder dysfunction due to injury to the nervous system, rather than due to direct injury to the bladder) and impotence.

In general, spinal cord transection anywhere in the cervical region would result in quadriplegia (sometimes referred to as tetraplegia). Sometimes a distinction is made between the term "quadriplegia," used to indicate total paralysis of all four limbs, and the term "quadriparesis," used to indicate partial loss of motion in all four limbs.

Cervical cord injuries can also affect the ability to breathe. The phrenic nerve, which controls the respiratory diaphragm (and hence the ability to breathe), is usually composed of a combination of nerve branches from the third, fourth, and fifth cervical levels. If the cord were severed above this level, the patient would be unable to breathe, and hence death would result.[8]

For several reasons, it is often difficult to define an exact level of spinal cord injury. First, more than one cord location may be injured. Second, lesions may affect the cord at a location remote from the original injury. For example, a hematoma may accumulate, due to gravity, below the actual vascular injury. As the hematoma grows, it then pushes against the cord or a spinal nerve and thereby causes injury at a second site. Third, an injury can change in severity over time. For example, in one clinical study, more than 90% of the patients showed an improvement of at least two sensory levels (e.g., C6 rather than C4) and approximately 30% of the patients showed an improvement of at least three sensory levels (Young 1989). (It should be emphasized that particularly for cervical injuries, a difference of two or three sensory levels is quite significant.)

Injuries to the spinal cord are not always complete and hence do not always produce complete loss of function and sensation below the level of injury. Quite the contrary, injuries to part of the cord are relatively common and produce what are referred to as incomplete spinal cord syndromes. Three incomplete syndromes, namely, central cord syndrome, anterior cord syndrome, and cord hemisection syndrome, account for more than 90% of all the incomplete cord syndromes (Hockberger 1988), and will be discussed here.

The cord's cross-sectional structure (viewed in a horizontal plane) may be described as a bow tie-shaped central section (the gray matter), surrounded by the peripheral white matter (Figures 1.6 and 1.24). The cord displays symmetry with respect to the mid-sagittal plane (left-right symmetry), and each half may be divided into anterior, lateral, and posterior regions (Figure 1.24).

Neural impulses going up to the brain have their own pathways—they are transmitted via bundles of nerve fibers called ascending tracts. Messages coming down from the brain have their own pathways, called descending tracts. Injury to a particular tract will interfere with the function associated with that tract.

One tract of interest is the lateral spinothalamic tract. This is an ascending pathway located in the lateral region (Figure 1.24) and contains most of the fibers that convey information to the brain regarding pain or temperature.

---

[8] An exception to this would be if the patient could be kept alive via artificial respiration until transported to a medical facility. The patient could then be ventilated mechanically, or helped to breathe on his/her own, with the assistance of a phrenic nerve pacer (similar to a heart pacemaker).

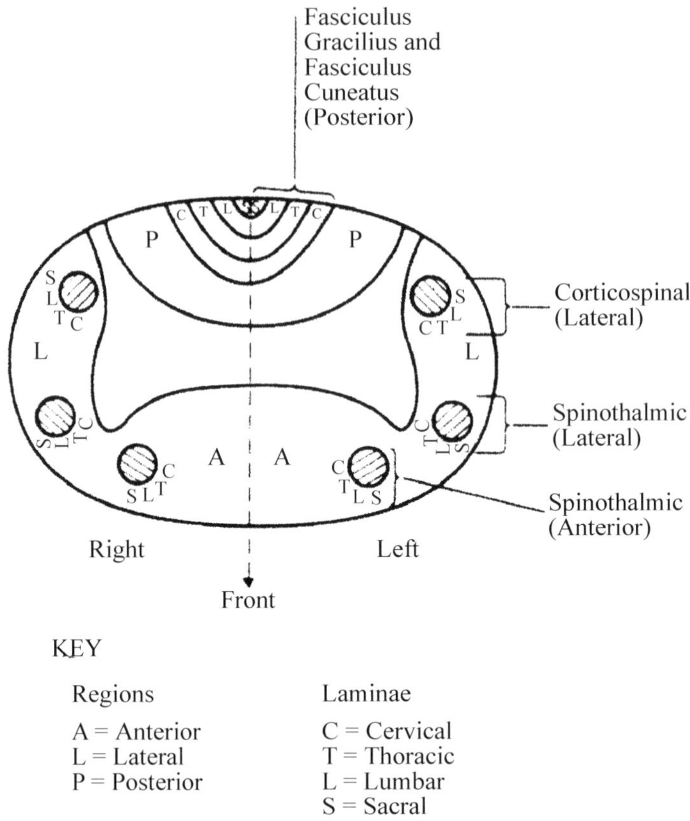

Figure 1.24   Lamination of spinal cord tracts.   [Reproduced with permission.   Source: Pike 1990.]

There are four other major tracts of interest for this discussion: the anterior spinothalamic tract, the lateral corticospinal tract, and the fasciculus gracilis and fasciculus cuneatus, usually referred to as the posterior tracts (Figures 1.24 and 1.25). The anterior spinothalamic tract is associated with light touch; the lateral corticospinal tract, limb movement; and the fasciculus gracilis and fasciculus cuneatus, or posterior tracts, proprioception (position), two-point tactile discrimination, and vibrational sensory information.

Within some of the tracts, the "wiring" has a laminar (i.e., layered) arrangement, with the longer layers being on the outside (i.e., more superficial). Thus, the sacral lamina, which connects the brain to the sacral region of the cord, is

SPINAL TRACT NAME AND FUNCTION (BY REGION)		
REGION	**NAME**	**FUNCTION**
ANTERIOR	**SPINO-THALMIC**	**TOUCH**
LATERAL	**SPINO-THALMIC**	**PAIN, TEMPERATURE (CONTRALATERAL)**
	CORTICO-SPINAL	**MOTOR**
POSTERIOR	**FASCICULUS GRACILIUS AND FASCICULUS CUNEATUS**	**POSITION, VIBRATION, TOUCH**

Figure 1.25 Spinal tract names and functions. [Reproduced with permission. Source: Pike 1990.]

the longest, and is on the outside. Beneath this is the next longest lamina, which goes from the brain to the lumbar region, followed by the thoracic lamina, and finally the cervical lamina, which is the innermost and the shortest. The "wires" carrying the pain and temperature signals in the lateral spinothalamic tract crossover in such a way that an injury to the right anterolateral cord region can produce loss of pain and temperature sensation on the left side (Figures 1.24 and 1.26). These anatomic and physiologic concepts can now be applied to specific cord injuries.

Central cord syndrome, as the name implies, refers to injury to the central (i.e., axial) part of the cord. Due to the laminar structure of some of the tracts of the cord, the more centrally located laminae of the anterior and lateral tracts are more likely to be affected. (The posterior tracts also have a laminar structure, but they do not have a deep-superficial arrangement, i.e., stacking of the layers is not oriented along a line going from the surface to the interior of the cord.) (Figures 1.24 and 1.27)

Central cord syndrome therefore results in loss mostly to the upper extremities (that is, it affects the cervical and thoracic laminae more than the lumbar and sacral laminae) (Figures 1.24 and 1.27), and results in impaired temperature and pain sensation (Figures 1.25 and 1.27). The seemingly contradictory

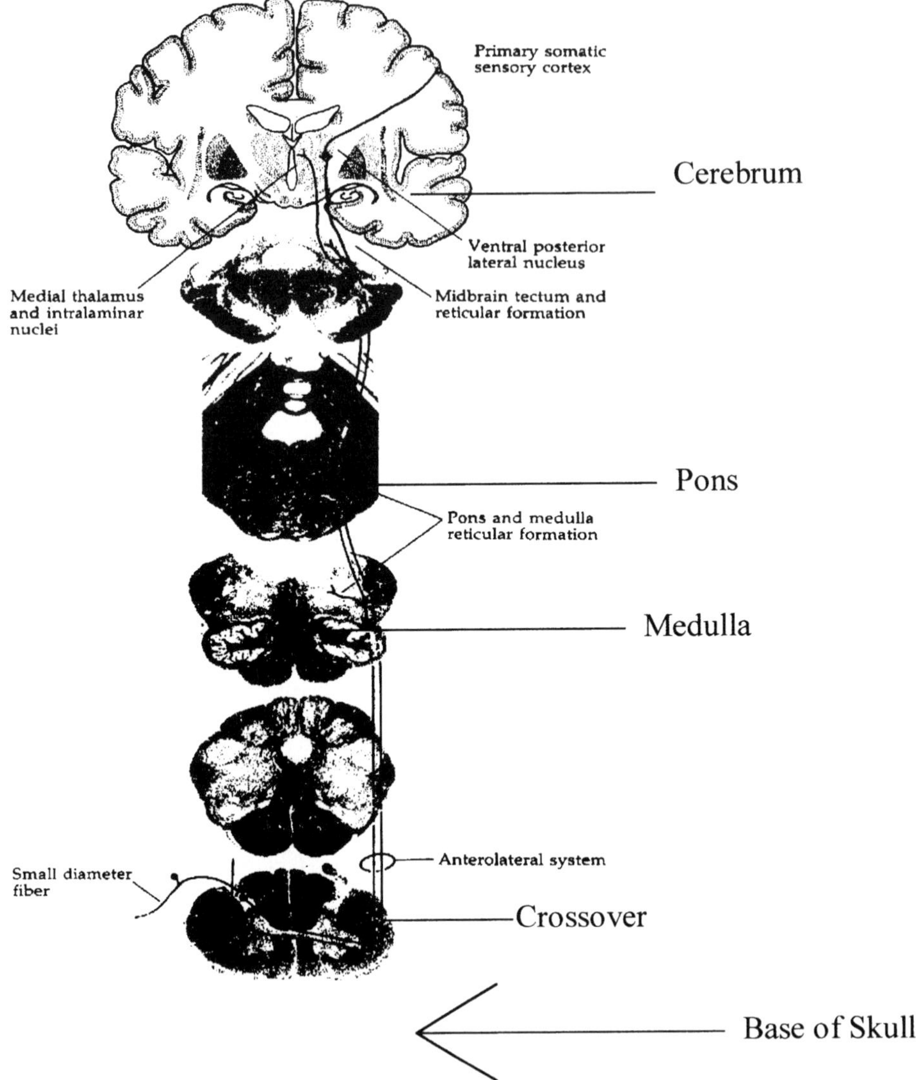

Figure 1.26 Cross-over of nerve fibers in spinal cord tract. [Reproduced with permission of The McGraw-Hill Companies. Source: Martin, J.H. Neuroanatomy: Text and Atlas. Elsevier (New York), 1989.]

FUNCTION	Syndrome and Function Affected		
	ANT.	**CENT.**	**HEMI**
TOUCH			X
PAIN, TEMPERATURE (CONTRALATERAL)	X	X	X
MOTOR	X (LOWER)	X	X
POSITION, VIBRATION, TOUCH			X X X

Figure 1.27 Spinal cord syndromes and tracts affected. [Reproduced with permission. Source: Pike 1990.]

effects of this injury, namely, loss of function associated with the cervical region of the cord, without loss of function associated with the lower cord (especially the sacral region), is sometimes referred to as sacral sparing.

Anterior cord syndrome may be somewhat misleadingly named, in that it typically involves injury to the lateral tract as well as to the anterior tract (Figures 1.24, 1.25, and 1.27). It produces loss mostly of lower extremity function and sphincter control (incontinence), and loss of pain and temperature sensation. Cord hemisection syndrome (Brown-Sequard syndrome) refers to injury to either the left or right half of the spinal cord. (Although Brown-Sequard classically refers to a syndrome affecting an entire half of the cord, in practice, partial Brown-Sequard is much more common.)

Not surprisingly, Brown-Sequard results in symptoms on one side. Perhaps surprisingly, however, all symptoms are not on the same side. That is, there is decreased or lost awareness of light touch, position and vibration sensations, and motor loss, on the same side of the body as the spinal cord injury (ipsilateral), but diminished sensation (e.g., awareness of temperature and pain) on the opposite side of the body (contralateral). Note that of the three syndromes discussed, only Brown-Sequard is likely to affect both the anterior spinothalamic tract and the posterior tracts, and hence only Brown-Sequard generally results in loss of touch sensation (Figures 1.24, 1.25, and 1.27).

It will be noted (Figure 1.25) that the anterior spinothalamic tract conveys sensory information. However, anterior cord syndrome does not have much effect on this function because the posterior tracts, which are unaffected, share this function. (A more detailed discussion of spinal cord anatomy may be found in a neuro-anatomy text, e.g., Martin 1989, or in a neuro-physiology text, e.g., Gilman 1982.)

The various deficits described here, which result from injury to only part of the spinal cord, help to explain why the classification of a spine fracture as stable or unstable is so important—although a stable spinal fracture may involve substantial injury, it is when the injury is unstable that there needs to be particular concern about the occurrence of *additional* cord injury.

After spinal trauma, a condition called spinal shock may exist. This refers to a transient condition, usually lasting no more than 24 hours and character-ized by a diminution or total loss of all reflexes below the site of injury (Bohlman 1986). Spinal shock must be distinguished from the long-term/permanent losses previously discussed. Also note that the spine might be distorted for an instant and then return to its normal position (spontaneously reduce). Thus, although at the time of examination the bony spine may "look fine" the brief distortion may have been sufficient to cause injury.

Spinal fracture and closed head injury (CHI) frequently occur together (Davidoff 1988; Baxt 1985). This is significant for several reasons. First, as the result of the head injury, the patient may not be able to describe, or may not even be aware of, the spinal injury. In addition, those providing medical treatment may need to first treat other injuries that pose a more immediate threat to life (e.g., head injuries). Furthermore, even after all injuries are assessed and treated, neurological deficits resulting from head injury may adversely affect the patient's ability to deal with the various medical, psycho-logical, and social morbidities of the spinal cord injury per se. Thus, these other factors may affect the long-term consequences without affecting the injuries per se. In addition to the loss of mobility and sensation, medical sequelae of spinal cord injury can include traumatic interruption of vaso-regulatory and thermo-regulatory function. The former may result in orthostatic hypotension (blood pressure suddenly drops when the person stands) and bradycardia (abnormally slow heartbeat), and the latter may result in poikilothermia (extremes of body temperature) (Baxt 1985).

Secondary effects may also include bladder and kidney infections, due to loss of proper emptying function for these organs, and decubitus ulcers (skin pressure sores), as the result of lengthy confinement to bed (either due to paralysis or other injuries that require bed rest). Decubitus ulcers, in turn, may become quite severe in their own right (Connolly 1988; Hunt 1988).

(Discussions of spinal injury mechanisms are also provided in Baxt 1985; Carroll 1988; Daffner 1996; D'Ambrosia 1986; Harris 1996; Helms 1989; Jeffreys 1993; Levine 1998; Levy 1986; Nightingale 1996; Mirvis 1992; Nahum 1993; Pike 2000; Resnick 1988; Rhea 1989; Levine 1998; White 1990; and Yoganandan 2000. A detailed discussion of the motor, sensory, and reflex losses associated with spinal cord lesions at each vertebral level is provided in Hoppenfeld 1977.)

ANTERIOR NECK INJURIES

Thus far, this chapter has discussed injury to the posterior region of the neck (vertebrae and associated structures), due primarily to head motion, with or without head impact. Another injury mechanism—injury to the anterior region of the neck due to neck impact—will now be discussed. As is indicated below, even seemingly modest injuries have the potential to become quite significant because of the role of neck structures in supplying blood to the brain and air to the lungs.

There are many important structures in the front of the neck, including the thyroid and cricoid cartilages, larynx, and trachea (Figures 1.28 and 1.29). Although these too may be injured via neck motion, they are also somewhat vulnerable to frontal impacts, especially if the neck is hyperextended. In particular, the thyroid cartilage (the Adam's apple) is in a prominent location (Figure 1.28) and has a low fracture force (typically less than 100 lb) (SAE 1986). Similar to injuries to other structures of the neck, cartilage fractures may not be especially significant in and of themselves, but because of their proximity to the airway and to the cerebral vasculature, they may produce interference with airway patency and/or carotid blood flow (blood supply to the brain).

The anterior structures of the neck may also be injured by neck motion, as well as by a variety of other injury mechanisms. For example, the trachea (Figure 1.29) may be injured by increased intra-tracheal pressure caused by chest compression or by a shearing injury due to chest compression. Or, perhaps somewhat surprisingly, a tearing injury may be produced by *lateral* movement of the lungs in response to *anterior-posterior* compression of the chest (from chest impact) (Hurst 1987). These and other neck injuries are discussed in Bland 1994; Camins 1992; Campbell 1988; Nolph 1987; Richardson 1987; Rosen 1988; Sabiston 1987; Sherk 1989; White 1990; and Yoganandan 2000.

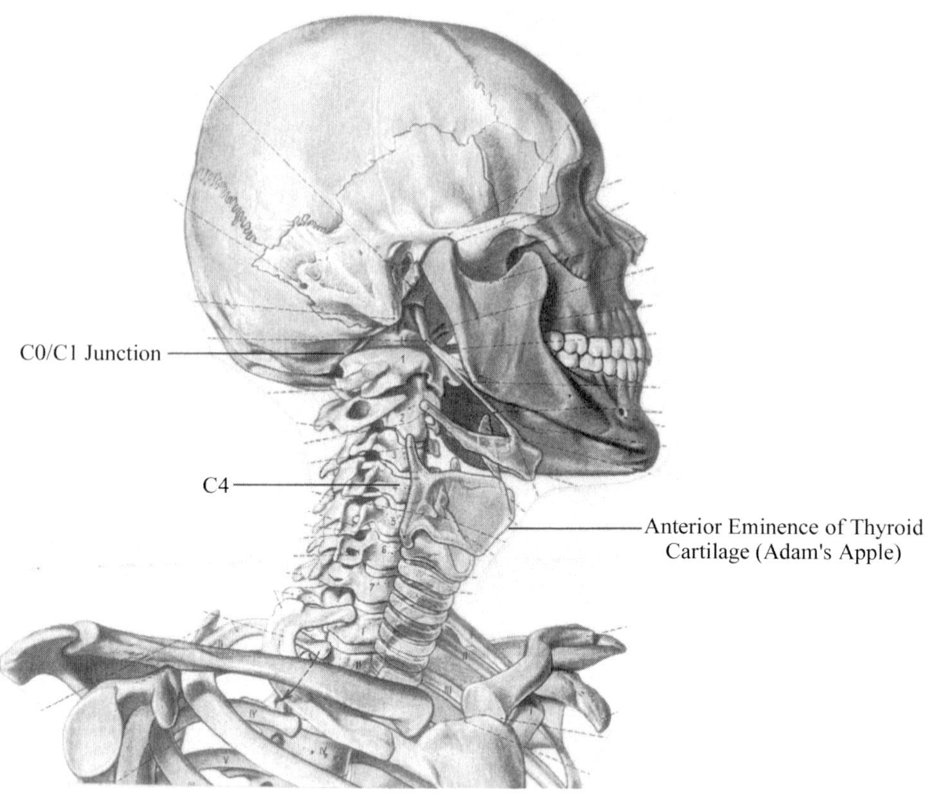

Figure 1.28   Skeleton, C0–T1, lateral view.   [Reproduced with permission.   Source: Pernkopf 1963.]

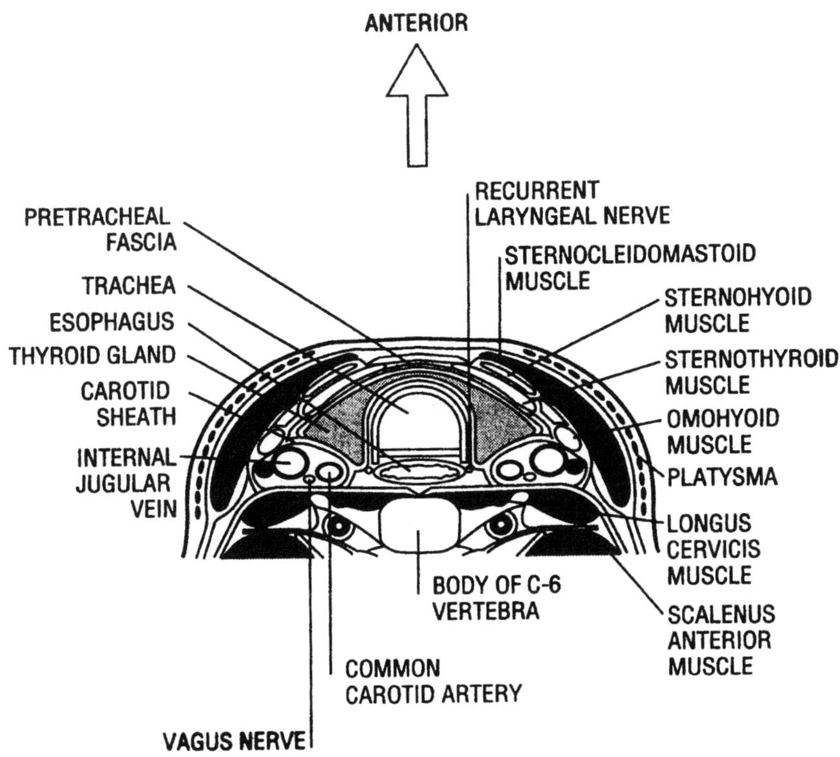

Figure 1.29 Anterior structures of the neck. [Reproduced with permission. Source: Pike 1990.]

Chapter 2

Imaging

JEFFREY A. PIKE
RONALD S. ADLER
RONALD MAIO
MARY ANN GREGOR

INTRODUCTION

Diagnostic imaging may be briefly defined as "a visual presentation of patient information which is used to help make a diagnosis." The image is usually based on information from the inside of the body; hence, much diagnostic imaging is based on information conveyed through non-visible energy, such as x-rays (Figure 2.1), which can pass through the skin and other structures. Furthermore, some diagnostic images convey information about the body's function rather than structure, and this information might not be visibly discernible even if the body were surgically "opened."

There are several ways of categorizing diagnostic imaging techniques. Perhaps the most common is based on the way the image is formed—that is, whether the energy used to generate the image is transmitted, reflected, or emitted by the body region (or structure) under investigation. Another way of categorizing diagnostic imaging techniques is by the type of information that the imaging technique provides—namely, structural or functional.

The following discussion emphasizes current methodologies and concepts that are most likely to be encountered when reviewing and analyzing medical records in conjunction with vehicle crash-related cervical trauma. In addition, this discussion is intended to serve as an introduction to the basic imaging concepts, which are likely to be the foundation for future developments. The discussion will focus on three imaging modalities: plain film radiography (x-rays), computed tomography (CT), and magnetic resonance imaging (MRI, or simply MR). In preparing this section, a great deal of effort was expended in obtaining films that were easy to read and that readily illustrated the points being made. One trade-off for this clarity, however, is that the films selected may not convey the range of image quality that is encountered (in the "real world") and the subtlety with which injuries may be depicted. This trade-off is appropriate, but is worthy of mention.

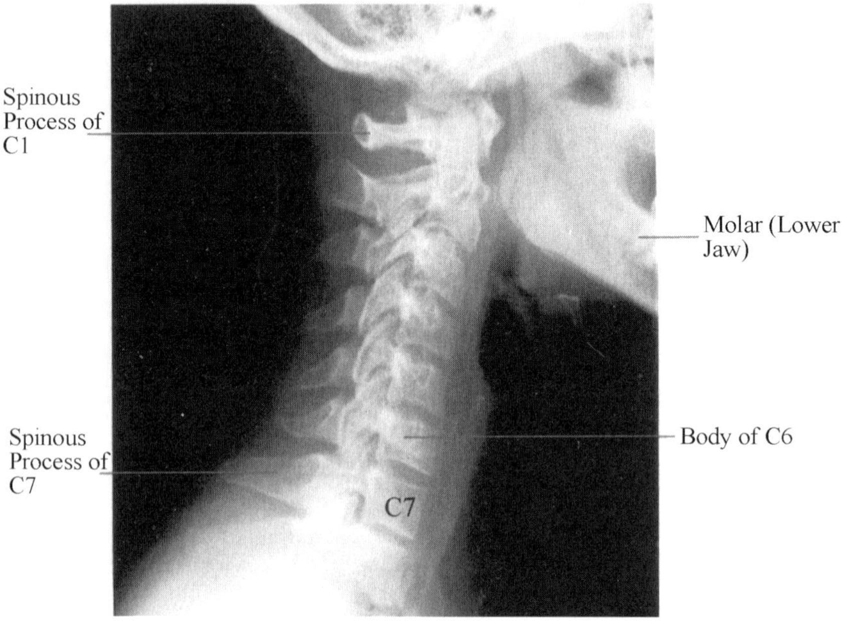

Figure 2.1   Radiograph (x-ray) of the neck (sagittal view).

BACKGROUND

Energy and Radiation

This section presents background material, with a goal of exploring some of the many factors that are weighed in deciding what is the best image for a given situation and some of the compromises involved in this decision. In this discussion, radiation or radiant energy will be used to refer to energy that disperses. This definition includes nuclear radiation, as well as x-rays, radio frequencies, and light.

One common way of classifying energy is by its wavelength (Figure 2.2). There is a continuum of wavelengths and within this continuum, various groupings (bands) of wavelengths that have similar properties have been identified. Wavelengths are specified in units of length, and the basic unit is the meter (approximately 39.4 inches). A unique frequency is associated with radiation of each wavelength, and so radiation may alternatively be characterized and grouped by its characteristic frequency. The basic unit of frequency is the hertz, which is defined as one cycle per second. A megahertz, abbreviated MHz, corresponds to one million cycles per second.

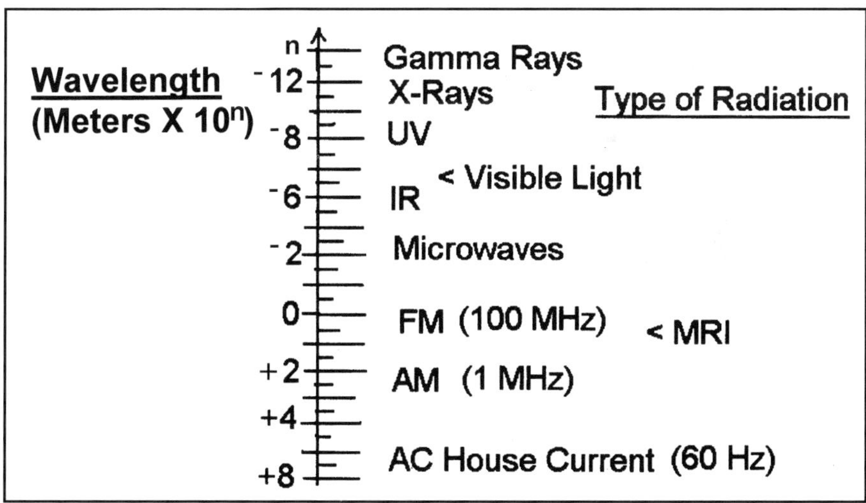

Figure 2.2 Electromagnetic spectrum (wavelengths and frequencies of electromagnetic radiant energy).

The relationship between wavelength, λ, in meters and frequency, f, in MHz, is given by the following equation:

$$f \times \lambda = 300$$

Thus, radiation with frequencies ranging from the middle of the AM radio band (approximately 1.0 MHz) to the middle of the FM radio band (approximately 100 MHz) corresponds to wavelengths ranging from 300 meters to 3 meters. (As will be discussed later, one of the imaging modalities, magnetic resonance [MR], causes structures within the body to emit radio frequency signals, and the MR equipment then creates visible images based on these signals.) Diagnostic imaging in a cervical trauma environment often utilizes radiation in the x-ray range (Figure 2.2).

Visible light has a much higher frequency than radio waves, and x-rays, in turn, have much higher frequency than visible light (Figure 2.2). The energy associated with a particular frequency determines how radiation of that frequency may be used to form images. For example, x-rays are used to form images by taking advantage of the way some of them will pass through the body, with more dense structures (e.g., bones) passing less of the entering radiation than structures that are less dense.[9]

X-Rays

X-rays used for diagnostic imaging are produced using an x-ray tube. Basically, the x-ray tube consists of two electrodes in a vacuum tube. The negative electrode, or filament, is made of high-resistance wire. Similar to the filament in a light bulb, the x-ray tube filament radiates energy when an electric current passes through it and causes it to heat up. In the case of the light bulb, much of the energy is in the visible range, and thus the process generates light. The x-ray filament, or cathode, however, emits electrons. These electrons are attracted to the oppositely charged electrode (the positive electrode or anode), and a high voltage differential is maintained between the anode and cathode to ensure that the electrons have a high velocity when they reach the anode. The anode is made of tungsten and emits x-rays each time one of the high-velocity electrons from the filament strikes it.

In the same way that light intensity and exposure time affect a regular (i.e., visible light) photograph, x-ray intensity and exposure time affect the exposure of x-ray film. The x-ray technologist (radiographer) controls film exposure by

---

[9] In this discussion, "dense" refers to radiodense, i.e., dense with respect to transmittal of x-rays and other electromagnetic radiation. To give some physical interpretation to radiodensity, this property increases with both increasing atomic number of the constituent elements of the structure and increasing thickness of the structure (Squire 1988).

varying the voltage and current used to generate the x-rays and the exposure time of the subject to the x-rays. These factors, in turn, contribute to the properties of the image, such as optical density, contrast, and detail.

Optical density may be simply defined as how dark an area appears to be when the developed x-ray film is viewed. A more radiodense structure appears lighter on a standard radiographic image, and a less radiodense structure appears darker. (This is similar to viewing a negative of regular photographic film—objects that are relatively dark when a print is made appear relatively light on the negative and vice versa.) Thus, the vertebrae appear rather light (Figure 2.1); they have a high physical density and produce an x-ray image of low optical density.

Contrast can then be defined as the relative (optical) densities of two adjacent areas—the greater the difference, the higher the contrast. Note that high-contrast images may represent a trade-off because very high-contrast images lose some information. All information is not equally useful, however, and the information loss may be quite acceptable if the improved contrast helps provide relevant information.

The electrical power delivered to an x-ray tube is the product of the voltage and the current; therefore, one might expect that these two quantities would contribute equally to image characteristics. This is not the case. Generally, a 15% increase in voltage will provide about the same increase in optical density as a doubling of the current (Bontrager 1993). Thus, it may seem that an obvious strategy to get the best image would be to maximize the voltage and minimize the current. However, increasing the voltage supplied to the x-ray tube decreases the contrast of the image. Thus, increasing the voltage increases the density, but at the expense of decreasing the contrast. Increasing the current increases the density of the image, but also exposes the patient to more radiation per image. Therefore, x-rays will usually be taken at the combination of highest voltage and lowest current that yields adequate exposure (Bontrager 1993).

Note that in practice, in x-ray imaging, the x-rays do not land directly on special x-ray sensitive film that is exposed by x-rays per se. Rather, the film (a regular, light-sensitive film) is packaged between two x-ray sensitive screens. The x-ray sensitive screens emit visible light when x-rays strike them, and the visible light from the screens then exposes the film. Such an arrangement is used because it requires less x-radiation than if the x-rays directly exposed the film. As will be discussed next, one negative aspect of such a system is that greater sensitivity is achieved at the expense of decreased resolution.

(Note that the trend is toward digital acquisition, i.e., having images entered directly into a computer, thereby eliminating "the middle man"—the film.)

In the following section on image quality, the detail of an image is a measure of how sharp (non-blurry) the image is. Blurriness is often introduced by the patient moving during imaging. Possible sources of movement, post neck trauma, include "voluntary" movement in response to injury-related pain or involuntary muscle spasm. If motion does introduce blurriness, supplemental x-rays may be taken, using a shorter exposure time or after an immobilization device is applied.

Image Quality

One factor that determines the particular imaging modality selected (i.e., whether it will be plain film, CT, or MRI) is which modality is likely to provide the highest-quality image. Although the phrase "image quality" can usually be interpreted as the degree of anatomic detail or anatomic fidelity, anatomic detail is not the goal per se—an image with enough fidelity to tell the physician what he or she needs to know may be preferable in other respects. For example, it may be faster. In many instances, the purpose of the imaging is to find out "what's wrong," and the utility of a given imaging modality is largely based on the extent to which the image it provides is able to help answer this question. (Of course, other factors, such as how quickly an image can be obtained, complications associated with the imaging procedure, and restrictions on usage, are also considered.)

It is important to note that the term "image quality" may be applied to an image that is physiologic rather than anatomic (and hence, anatomic fidelity would not apply). For example, a bone scan is used to indicate the general location of a pathological condition, rather than the exact location or nature of the pathology (Figure 2.3). Indeed, bone scans are useful in the case of occult fractures—fractures that are suspected but have not yet been located. In such cases, the bone scan can serve as a preliminary screen, to indicate the number and approximate location of occult fractures (if any).

Two important aspects of image quality are spatial resolution and contrast. Spatial resolution refers to how small of an object may be depicted (or how much detail is obtainable for a given subject). Contrast, on the other hand, refers to how well the object of interest may be distinguished from adjacent objects. We also may refer to the "contrast range" of a particular image. To understand this concept, it helps to consider the following analogy: Suppose

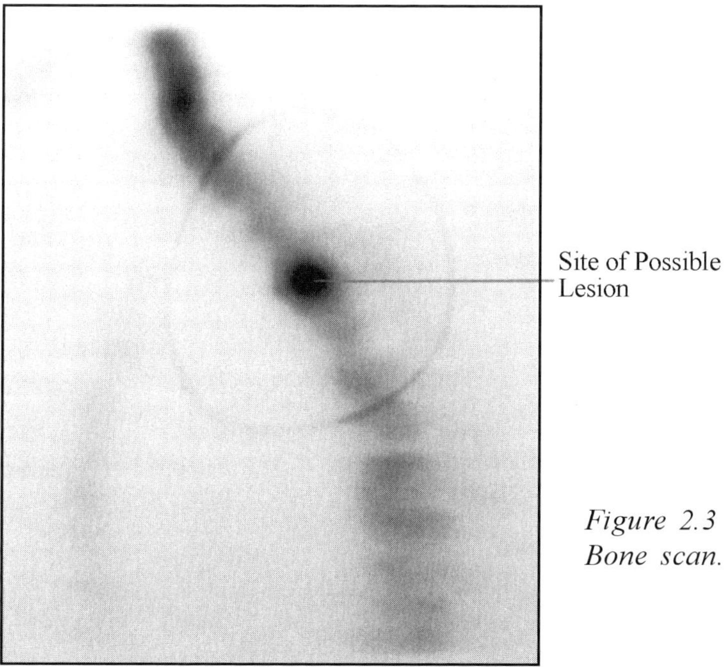

Figure 2.3
Bone scan.

we are using an optical camera and film to photograph a scene with both very high and very low levels of illumination (i.e., very light and very dark objects such as a plane flying in front of the sun). Under such conditions, we must decide if we want the film exposed to show details of the plane, in which case the sun would appear washed out (overexposed), or to show the sun as it actually appears, in which case the plane would appear dark (underexposed) and some detail would be lost. In such a case, the range of contrast of the subjects is too great for the film to show both the plane and the sun properly exposed. Similarly, diagnostic images must be adjusted to ensure the best possible exposure (and hence the best resolution) for the structure of interest. For example, a diagnostic image can be adjusted to optimize exposure for bones (or at least to expose them as best as possible), but at the expense of not providing optimum exposure for other structures (e.g., soft tissues). An image such as a CT image, which is adjusted to best display bone at the expense of other tissues, is often referred to as a bone window (Figure 2.4). In such an image, the other structures would appear too light or too dark. In either case, the image would not convey maximum information about these other structures.

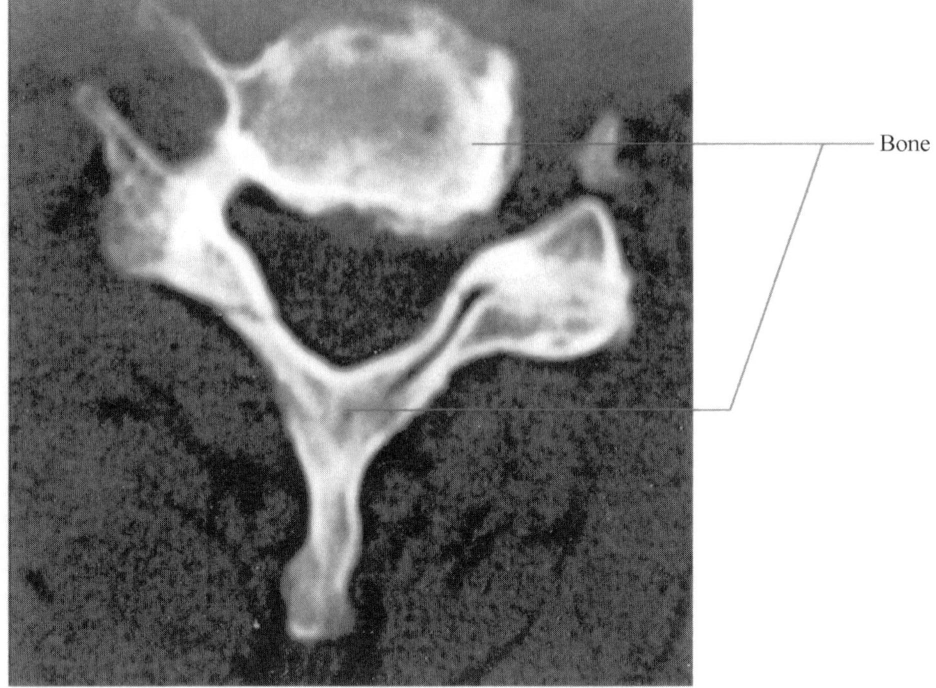

Figure 2.4   Bone window, computed tomography.

There are several approaches to improving contrast, including selecting a particular imaging modality based on the type of image required, increasing the radiation level, modifying the display to better expose the tissue of interest (e.g., obtaining a bone window), and introducing a dye (i.e., injecting the patient with a contrast medium) to enhance contrast, usually by darkening the image of the structure of interest. Increasing the radiation level has the drawback of exposing the subject to additional radiation. In addition, increased radiation may improve contrast at the expense of decreased sharpness.[10] Adjusting the exposure for the structure of interest has the drawback of providing reduced information about other structures. In addition, there are limits to how much improvement this may provide.

---

[10] The longer exposure means the image will be more susceptible to blurring due to occupant movement. In a neck trauma environment, movement may occur due to a variety of causes, including breathing, response to post-trauma pain, or associated head trauma, which may cause involuntary movement (Davidoff 1988; Pike 1990).

Under some circumstances, losing some structures on a diagnostic image may not only be acceptable, but may even be desirable. Indeed, loss of some structures can be used as a means to enhance contrast. Such an approach would seek to produce an image that does not include the "unimportant" structures, or includes them but greatly de-emphasizes them compared to the structure of interest. One way of achieving this is by adjusting the image so that surrounding structures appear washed out. (An example, discussed earlier, is the bone window—an image that emphasizes bone while de-emphasizing other substances such as air and blood.)

Introducing a contrast medium that has an affinity for the structure of interest may also increase contrast. Through the use of a contrast medium, one is able to produce a darker image of the structure of interest. One example of this approach is the angiogram (Figure 2.5).

In an angiogram, contrast may be further enhanced by using a computer to digitally subtract a "before" image (i.e., without dye) from an "after" image (i.e., with dye). An example of this is digital subtraction angiography (DSA),

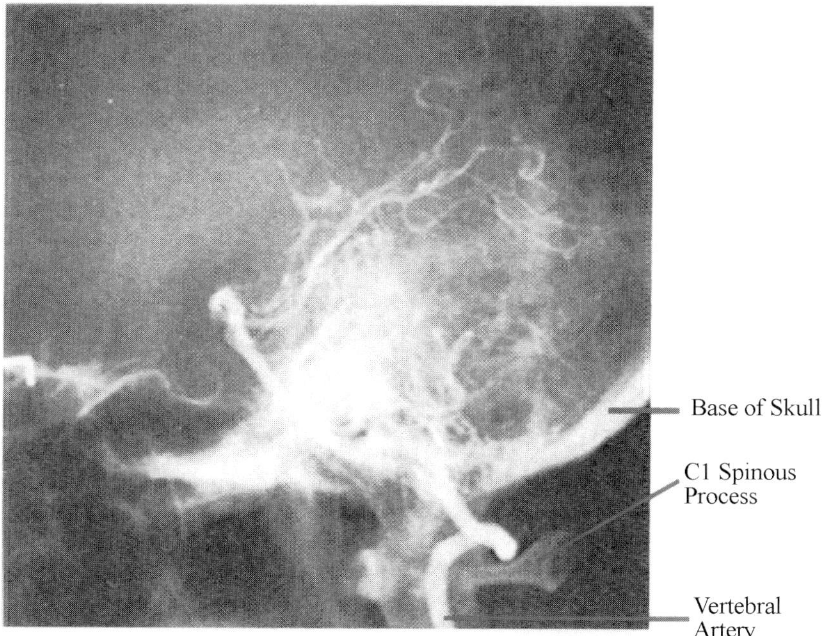

Figure 2.5 Angiogram. [Reproduced with permission. Source: Bontrager 1993]

where a die is injected into an artery or vein, a photo is taken before and after the dye's administration, and then the "before" photo is subtracted from the "after" photo to produce an image in which the surrounding soft tissue and bone have been removed. In a trauma setting, angiography is largely being replaced by CT. Angiography is still used in a trauma setting, however, especially to diagnose or assess vascular injury (Rhea 1988).

Digital subtraction angiography provides a good example of the types of trade-offs that are constantly being made in diagnostic imaging. Even the dyes formulated specially for diagnostic imaging produce some additional risk, so new developments that seek to minimize this risk are occurring constantly. One way to minimize the risk is to reduce the amount and/or change the type of contrast material needed to obtain the required image quality. (DSA requires a lower concentration of contrast medium than regular angiography.) Thus, a technique may be modified as the ability to enhance images by computer improves, such that less contrast or detail may be required in the original image.

Although contrast media may improve the visibility of some structures, like the window approach, contrast media may make other structures less visible. This brings with it the risk that one of the masked structures may in fact be important, e.g., a contrast agent may mask hemorrhage (Orrison 1989). In addition to degrading some aspects of image quality, contrast agents may produce undesirable "side effects" on the person being imaged. Although side effects are relatively rare (Oyesiku 1990) (frequency of approximately 5%) and most are mild, serious reactions (e.g., severe decrease in blood pressure) sometimes occur. Procedures such as DSA can cause complications (e.g., hematoma) at the injection site or remote from the injection site. Systemic complications can range from hives to cardiovascular collapse and kidney failure. The reported fatality rate due to contrast agent usage ranges from 1 in 14,000 to 1 in 70,000 (Rhea 1988).

The trade-off of improved image quality (and presumably improved diagnostic capability) versus possible undesirable side effects is made on an individual basis. This is due in part to the fact that certain segments of the population are at relatively high risk for some of the complications but not for others. For example, patients already having poor kidney function may be at special risk for kidney failure.

A nemesis of good image quality is "noise" (analogous to the static one hears when listening to an audio recording). For the purpose of this discussion, noise will be defined as anything that appears in the image but was not actually present. Because the goal of diagnostic imaging usually is image fidelity, it would seem that less noise is better. However, one of the most important aspects of these three factors—resolution, contrast, and noise—is that in general, any change in imaging that intensifies one of these factors (i.e., more resolution, more contrast, or less noise) does so at the expense of degrading at least one of the others.

Another imaging technique in which structures that are not of primary interest are subtracted is tomography. As will be discussed later in this chapter, tomography has widespread use in the diagnosis of blunt cervical trauma.

Analysis and Interpretation

Two important aspects of image analysis and interpretation are: (1) "finding what's there" (e.g., a fracture) and (2) determining "what isn't there" (e.g., to be able to say that the neck has no fractures). Sometimes, a fracture or other injury will be found when in fact none exists (a "false positive" error), and sometimes a fracture or other injury will be missed (a "false negative" error).

Difficulties in interpreting radiographs may be due to a variety of sources, including the presence of congenital or developmental abnormalities, superimposition of other structures, variations of normal anatomy, and limitations of the imaging system. A number of conditions may give the appearance of fractures even though no fracture is present.

An example of a false positive is illustrated in Figure 2.6. In this instance, there appears to be a fracture at the base of the dens, but this fracture line is actually the superimposition of the base of the atlas (and is referred to as the Mach effect). Another example of a false positive can occur when the neural foramen may be partially blocked by bone, but rather than it being a fracture fragment, it may be bone growth (osteophyte) due to a degenerative bone condition (Figure 2.7).

An easy way to categorize cervical spine injury is according to the type of tissue affected, and an easy way to categorize the tissue is as hard or soft. For this discussion, we will use the term "hard tissue" to refer to bone and "soft tissue" to refer to all other tissue—including ligaments, muscles, blood vessels, intervertebral discs, spinal nerves, and the spinal cord. (The soft tissue may also be subdivided into neural and non-neural, and this will be done when it benefits the discussion.) This is a useful distinction in terms of the types of injuries the different structures present and in terms of images often emphasizing one type of tissue over another. On x-rays, for example, a bone fracture may be indicated directly by the presence of a fracture line (Figure 2.8). In

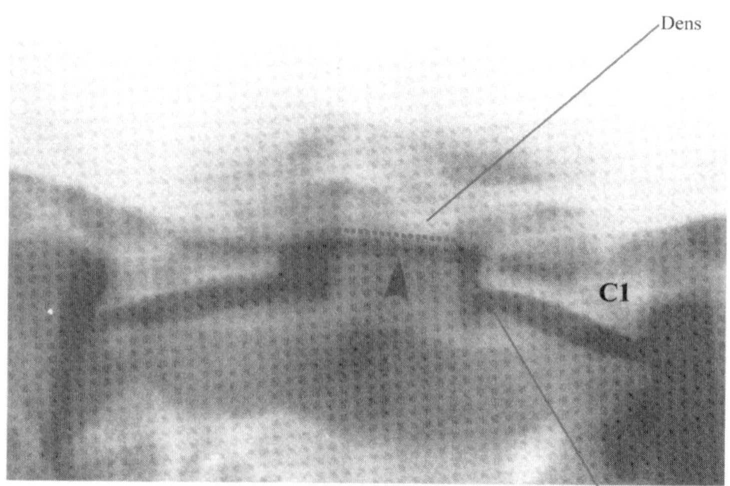

Figure 2.6   False (artifact) fracture on radiograph (Mach effect). [Reproduced with permission.   Source: Harris, J.; Mirvis, S. Radiology of Acute Cervical Spine Trauma, *3rd Edition. Williams & Wilkins (Baltimore), 1996.]*

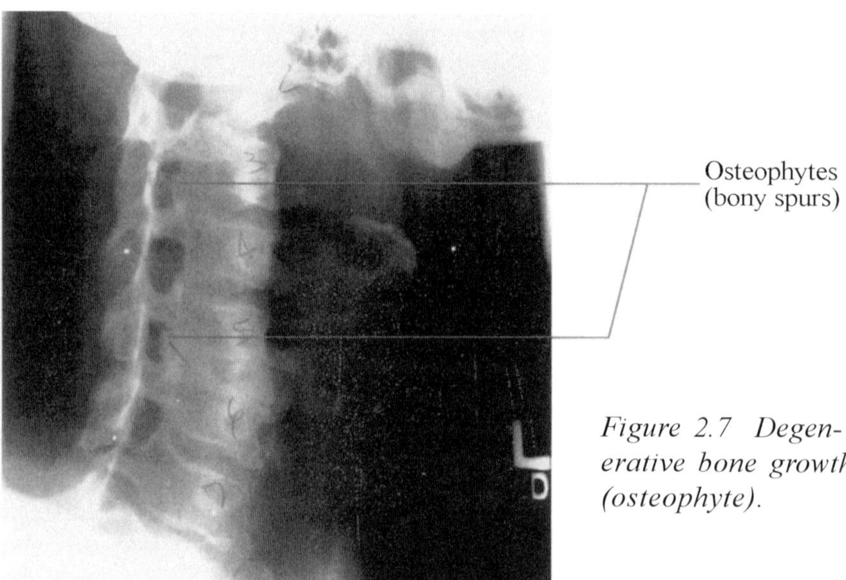

Figure 2.7   Degenerative bone growth (osteophyte).

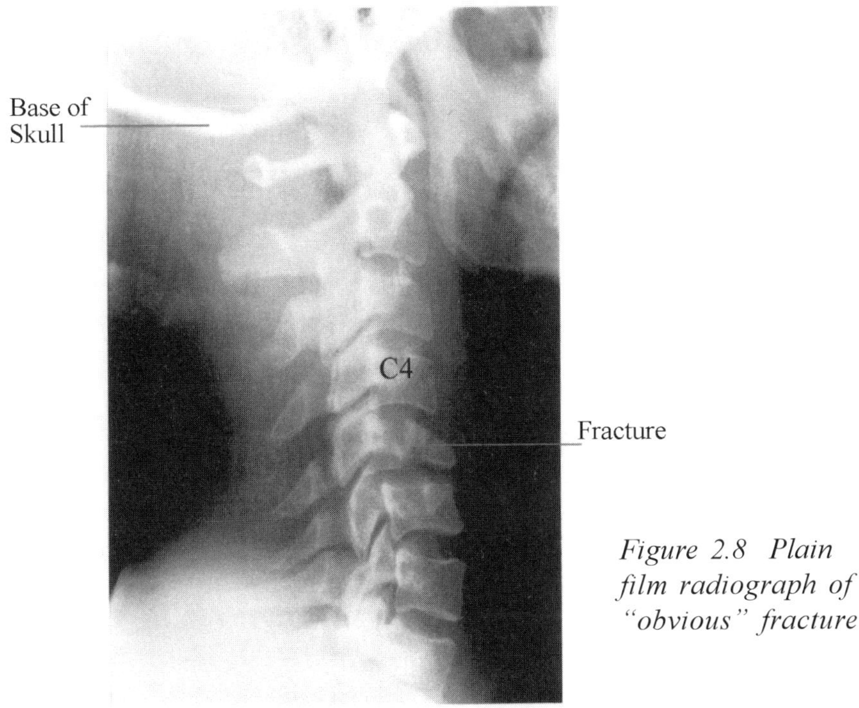

Figure 2.8 Plain film radiograph of "obvious" fracture.

contrast, many soft tissue injuries (e.g., ligament injuries) are not readily observable directly on x-rays and therefore must be indirectly deduced.

Possible indirect indications observable on x-rays include vertebral displacement (Chapter 3) and the accumulation of fluid (e.g., edema, accumulated blood). Accumulated fluid appears in an image as pre-vertebral swelling, i.e., the accumulated fluid produces an expansion of the soft tissue in front of the vertebrae. In the neck, the pharynx in front and the vertebrae behind bound the soft tissue; therefore, pre-vertebral swelling is also referred to as "retro-pharyngeal" swelling. A subtle fracture also may not be readily discernible on an x-ray, but similar to soft tissue injury, its presence sometimes may be detected indirectly by the presence of pre-vertebral swelling (Figure 2.9).

Soft tissue injury, including injury to ligaments, discs, and blood vessels, should not be considered any less important or any less potentially disabling than vertebral fractures. Quite the contrary, soft tissue injuries may be more severe, especially with regard to increased susceptibility to additional (post-crash) neurological injury. For example, an injury may involve the complete

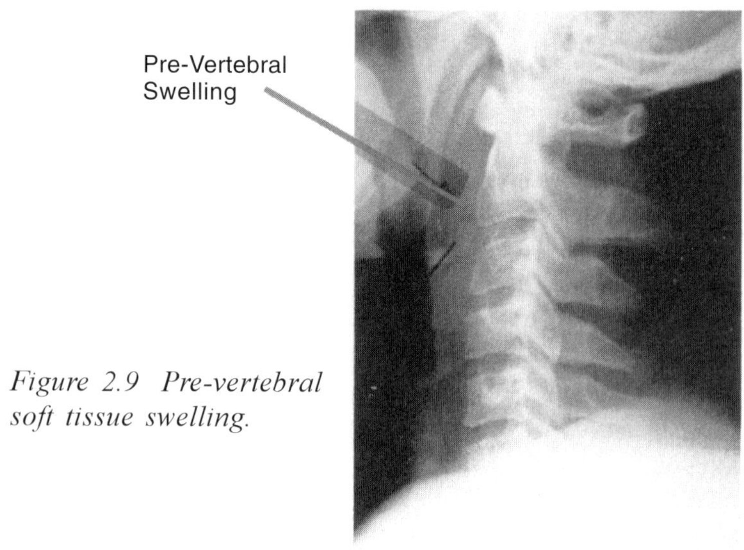

Figure 2.9   Pre-vertebral soft tissue swelling.

disruption of an intervertebral disc and complete disruption of the various ligaments that help hold the vertebrae in place. This, in turn, would mean that vertebrae adjacent to this section of the spine would be able to move with respect to each other and therefore might do so as the result of a very minor additional trauma, or even during regular everyday activity. This bony movement, in turn, could possibly produce spinal cord injury and result in paralysis.

An important innovation in x-ray imaging permits viewing a "slice" of the subject, rather than the traditional view of the entire depth. Such an image is called a tomogram. Tomograms were invented about 50 years ago but were generated by mechanical means until the early 1970s, when the first tomogram was produced using computer technology. Today, computed tomography (CT) is quite common.

A more recent innovation (1980s), called magnetic resonance imaging (MRI or MR), does not even use x-rays. Indeed, one of its most desirable features is thought to be that it uses only lower-frequency, lower-energy (non-ionizing) radiation. (Figure 2.2).[11] The radio waves used in MR diagnostic imaging do

---

[11] A discussion of wavelength, frequency, and energy may be found in an introductory physics text. A more detailed discussion of these concepts, specifically as they relate to MRI, may be found in a "physics of radiology" text, such as Bushong 1988, Hendee 1992, or Sorenson 1987.

not produce an image by passing through the body region of interest (the neck); rather, they are caused to be emitted from within the neck. This technique of obtaining images is referred to as emission, as compared to transmission for x-ray generated images.

PLAIN FILM RADIOGRAPHS (X-RAYS)

The lateral view shown (Figures 2.1 and 2.10) is an example of a "no-frills" x-ray and is often referred to as a "plain film." This film is a two-dimensional representation of a three-dimensional structure and so may also be thought of as a plane [sic] film. A plain film does not display information regarding depth and hence cannot provide a complete picture of the structure being imaged. In addition, a plain film may not indicate where along the length of the x-ray beam a lesion of interest is located, and it may not indicate the presence of an abnormality in the plane of the x-ray beam projection. Thus, it is often useful to take plain films from more than one view.

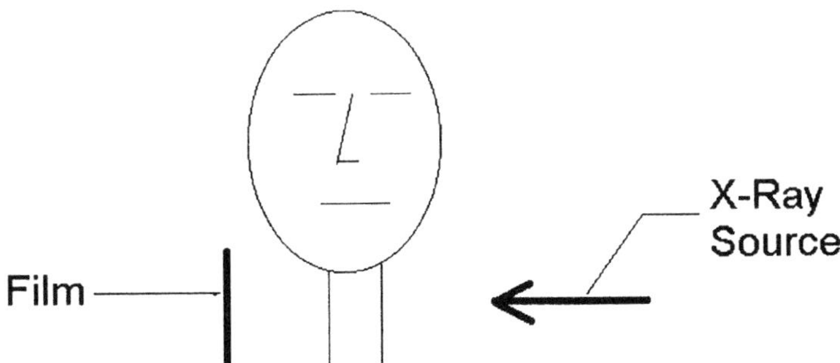

Figure 2.10. Positioning of x-ray source, body region of interest, and film for plain film radiograph (cross-table lateral view).

VARIOUS PLAIN FILM RADIOGRAPH VIEWS

As mentioned, plain film x-rays (radiographs) are often taken from more than one perspective or view. One or more parameters may be used to specify a particular x-ray view. These parameters include those used to specify the body region or sub-region being imaged (e.g., the odontoid view) (Figures 2.11 and 2.12) and the orientation of the x-ray beam with respect to the body

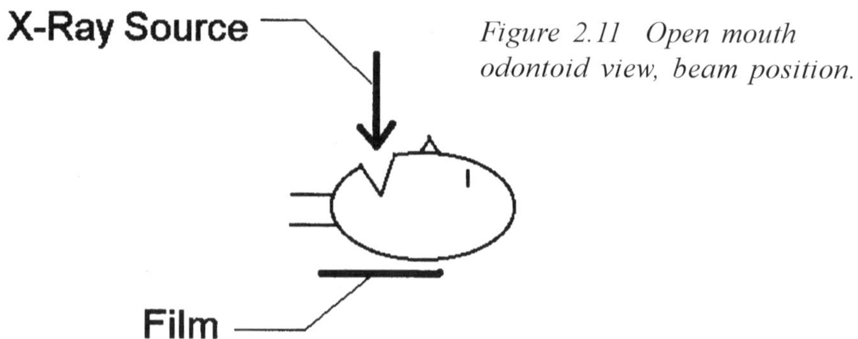

Figure 2.11 Open mouth odontoid view, beam position.

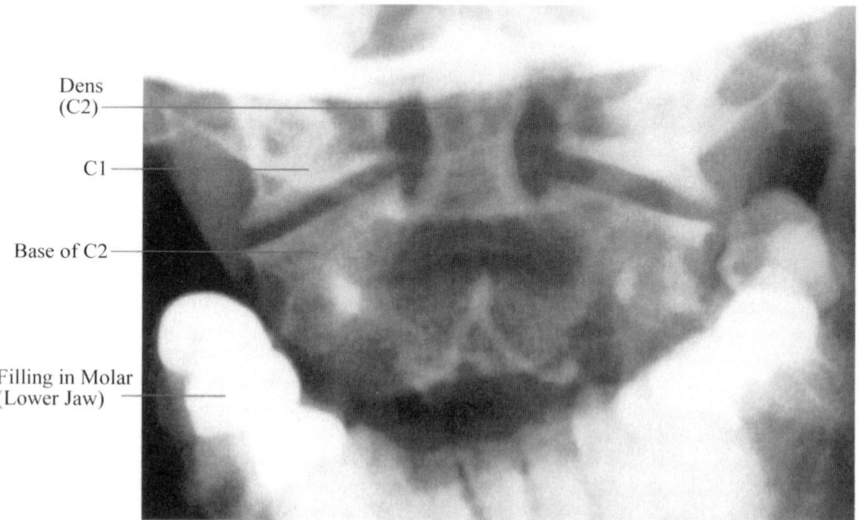

Figure 2.12 Open mouth odontoid view, radiograph.

(e.g., the oblique view) (Figures 2.13 and 2.14). The relative orientation of the body and the x-ray beam and to some extent the position of the internal structures of the body depends in part on the orientation of the body, e.g., whether the subject is standing or lying down. For the purpose of this discussion, it will be assumed that the subject is supine, i.e., lying on his/her back. (Exceptions will be indicated.)

In addition to the body region or sub-region being imaged and the orientation of the x-ray beam with respect to the body, the name of the view may also

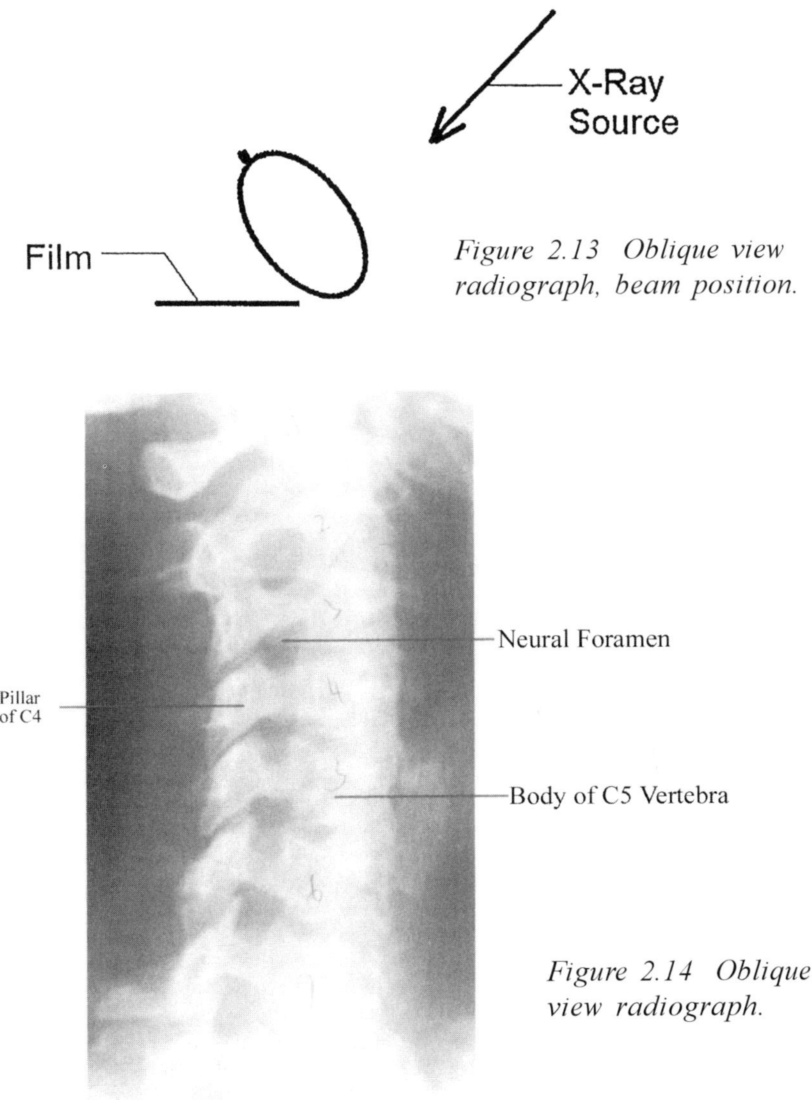

Figure 2.13 Oblique view radiograph, beam position.

Figure 2.14 Oblique view radiograph.

specify the direction of the x-ray beam, i.e., whether it is going from the subject's front to the subject's back, or vice versa. This distinction may be important because the part of the body where the x-ray exits is closest to the film and therefore is emphasized on the image. For example, an anteroposterior projection (A-P view) describes a configuration where the x-ray beam goes from the subject's anterior to the subject's posterior. Thus, the x-ray source is located in front of the subject, the x-ray film is located behind the subject (Figure 2.15), and the resulting radiograph will provide a better image of the posterior region than of the anterior region (Figure 2.16).[12] Conversely, if the front of the neck is of more interest, a posterior anterior projection (P-A view) may be selected.

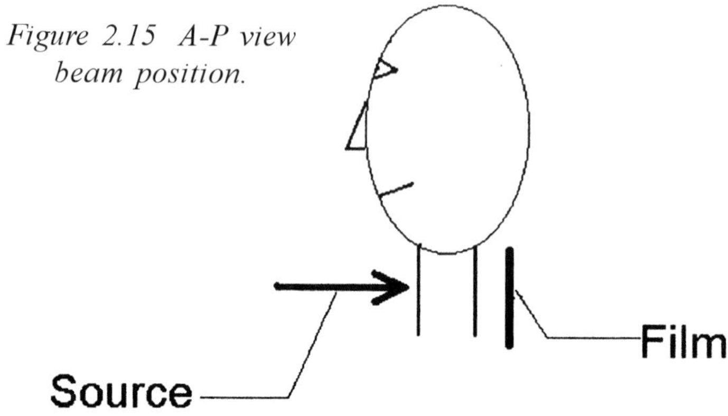

A separate convention is usually followed when describing lateral views—they are named for the side closest to the film, e.g., if the right side is closest to the film, the view is often referred to as a right lateral view. The lateral view may also be more fully specified, e.g., as a right posterior lateral, for a view with the x-ray source in front of the patient and the film near the right posterior of the patient.

In cases of neck trauma or suspected neck trauma, the lateral view is often taken first and is frequently supplemented with at least one other view (most commonly the A-P view). Lateral views, especially in a trauma environment, are often obtained with the patient lying supine (face up) rather than standing upright. If the patient is supine during the imaging, the lateral view is referred to as a cross-table lateral (CTL) view. If the imaging is conducted with the patient either sitting or standing, it is referred to as an erect lateral view.

---

[12] In some instances, the term "view" may be used to refer to only the radiographic image obtained from a particular x-ray path and not the path itself (in which case, the path is referred to as the projection) (Bontrager 1993). For the purpose of this discussion, the term "view" will be used to refer to the image, the path, or both. A distinction will be made if necessary.

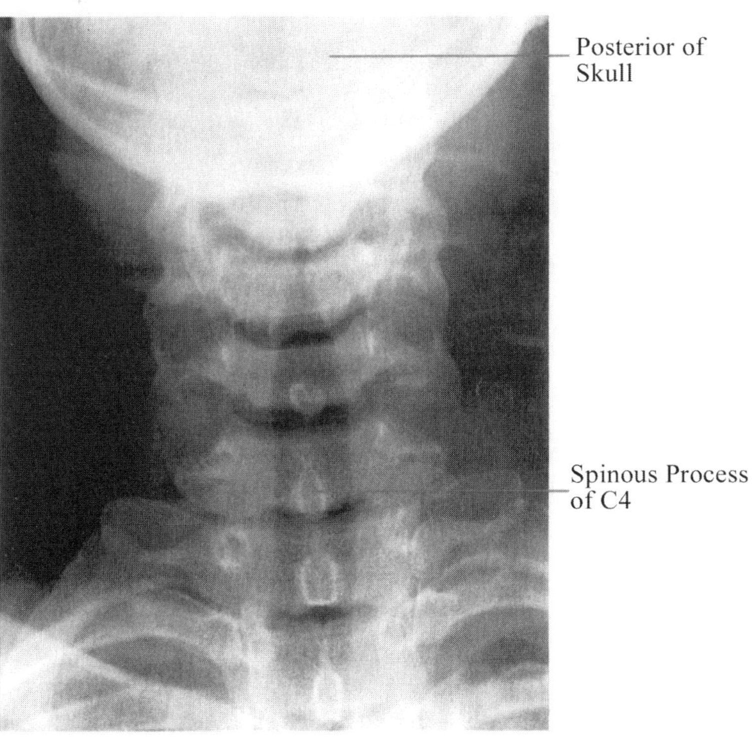

Figure 2.16 A-P view radiograph.

A minimal set of plain film radiographs (often CTL plus A-P views) is often used for screening, i.e., to determine if neck restraints such as cervical collars can be removed and if the neck can be moved to conduct other imaging. However, the basic set may prove diagnostic (i.e., may indicate a specific pathology), in which case additional views may not be obtained.

One of the goals of the initial imaging frequently is to "clear" the cervical spine, and medical records may include the notation "C-spine cleared" or "Cervical spine cleared" (Figure 2.17). The sample provided in Fig. 2.17 indicates the cervical spine had no fractures and was cleared by "Dr. ———." Basically, when the cervical spine is cleared, it means that at some point during the patient's early care, a health care provider (generally a physician) decided that the nature and extent of cervical injury has been adequately assessed to determine that the patient will not be at any appreciable risk of additional cervical injury from ordinary neck movement. Two important consequences of a cleared spine are that precautions such as neck immobilization (e.g., neck brace) may be discontinued and that the patient may move his or her neck as required (e.g., flexion, extension) to have additional images taken. Thus, notation that the cervical spine is cleared does not indicate that there is no neck injury—only that there is no injury that is severe enough to require neck immobilization or that would preclude the patient from trying voluntary neck movement.

Based on the patient's condition and the information (or lack thereof) provided by the initial views, lateral and A-P views may be supplemented with one or more of the following: odontoid (open mouth), oblique, pillar, swimmer, and flexion-extension views.

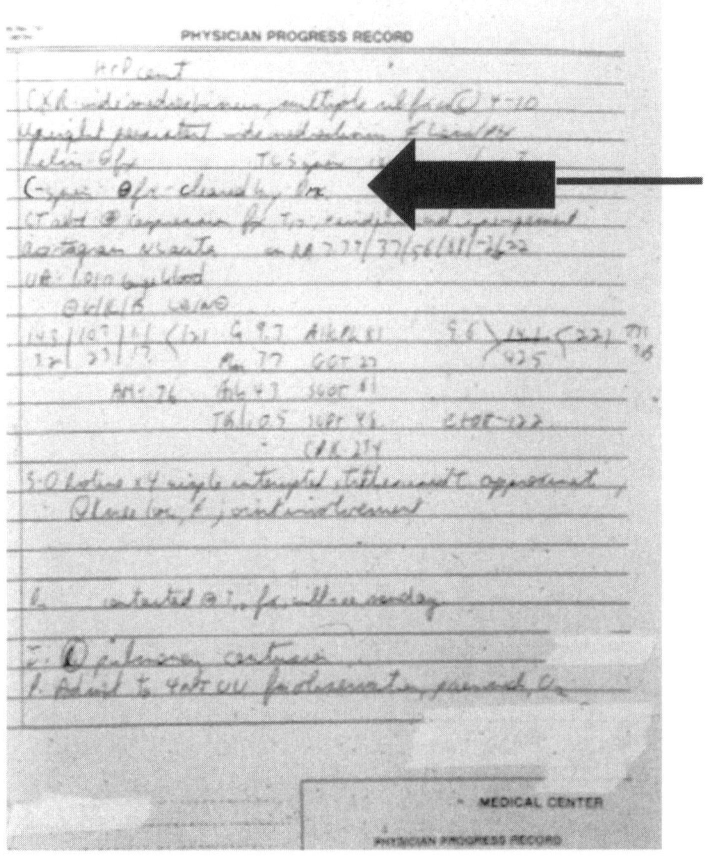

Figure 2.17 C-spine "cleared."

Cross-Table Lateral View (CTL)

A lateral view is usually the first neck x-ray taken and frequently provides the most information. This image may be obtained with the subject upright or supine, depending on the subject's condition. After trauma, the lateral view is frequently obtained with the patient supine and often in a cervical collar. In this position, the x-ray source is on one side of the table and the film on the other side (Figure 2.10), so the x-ray beam is essentially horizontal. To distinguish this lateral view from one obtained with the patient upright, the supine view is called the cross-table lateral view. Or, more formally, the upright view is called the erect lateral view, and the supine view is called the supine horizontal-beam lateral view.[13] The reason for distinguishing between these two views is that the orientation of the patient—whether supine or upright—may provide the clinician with relevant information. The patient's orientation can affect the influence of gravity on the position of various body structures and on blood flow.

The mnemonic "ABC'S" provides a framework for organizing the different features that are examined, namely, <u>A</u>lignment, <u>B</u>ones, <u>C</u>artilage, and <u>S</u>oft tissue space. Many of these features can be conceptualized by drawing a series of curves superimposed on the cervical vertebrae, and checking these curves for parallelism and continuity. As will be discussed, all curves should be smooth and generally parallel, and the lack of these traits can be indicative of various injuries. In effect, this procedure checks the alignment of the vertebrae and the integrity of the associated ligaments, blood vessels, and neural tissue.

The six curves (Figure 2.18) drawn on lateral views of the cervical spine will now be discussed. Curve 1 refers to the "S" (soft tissue) in the "ABC'S" mnemonic and will be discussed in a later section, titled "Soft Tissue Swelling." The remaining five curves (Curves 2 through 6) are used to study the alignment of the cervical vertebrae. Misalignment may be indicative of ligament tears, vertebra fracture, or relative displacement of one vertebra with respect to an adjacent vertebra—any of which may be indicative of neurological injury or the potential for neurological injury.

---

[13] If the lateral view does not adequately display the lower cervical spine (including the C7/T1 disc space), it may be supplemented with a modified CTL. The modified CTL involves applying manual traction to the shoulders by pulling down on the forearms (with the patient's arms at his or her side), to extend the upper extremities and lower the shoulders. Such traction cannot be applied to all patients and even when applied, may not produce the desired image, i.e., one without any blockage. Various "clues" regarding the location and nature of cervical spinal trauma are discernible from the CTL view.

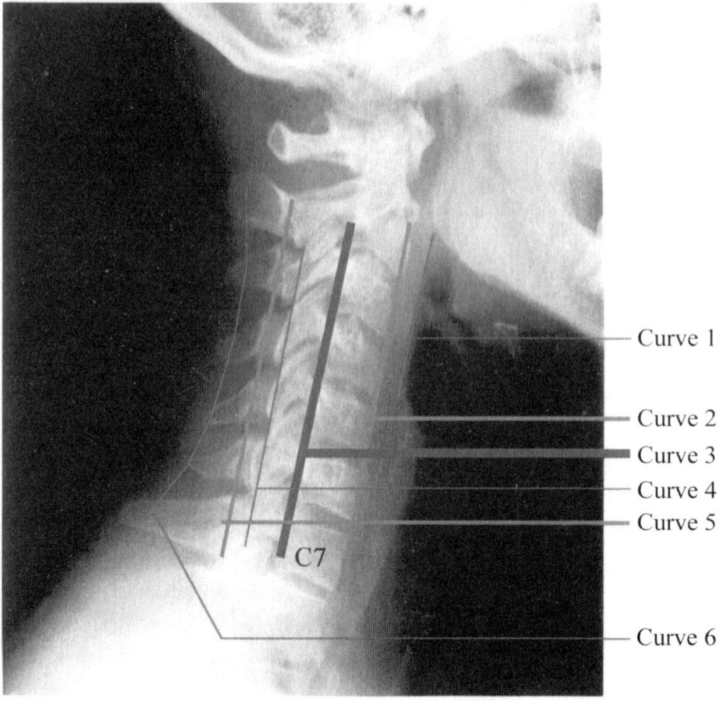

Figure 2.18   Lateral spinal view—six curves of alignment.

Alignment

The line labeled "Curve 2," the anterior vertebral body line (Figure 2.19), basically corresponds to the anterior longitudinal ligament (ALL) (Chapter 1). A disruption in the smoothness of this curve corresponds to a tear or rupture of the ligament (Figure 2.20) and an associated vertebral displacement.

Similarly, the line labeled "Curve 3," the posterior vertebral body line (Figure 2.21), corresponds to the posterior longitudinal ligament. Here, a disruption in the curve corresponds to a tear or rupture of the ligament and an associated vertebral displacement (Figure 2.22). Curves 2 and 3 should be essentially parallel and even a small offset—typically 3 mm—is suggestive of disruption of either one or both of the ligaments (ALL and PLL).[14] Similarly,

---

[14] Much of this discussion applies to the lower cervical vertebrae, C3 through C7. Regarding C1 and C2, the odontoid process (dens) of C2 is usually held in close approximation to the anterior arch of C1 by the transverse ligament. A separation of more than 3 mm (Straub 1989) between the anterior edge of the dens and C1 may indicate disruption of this ligament.

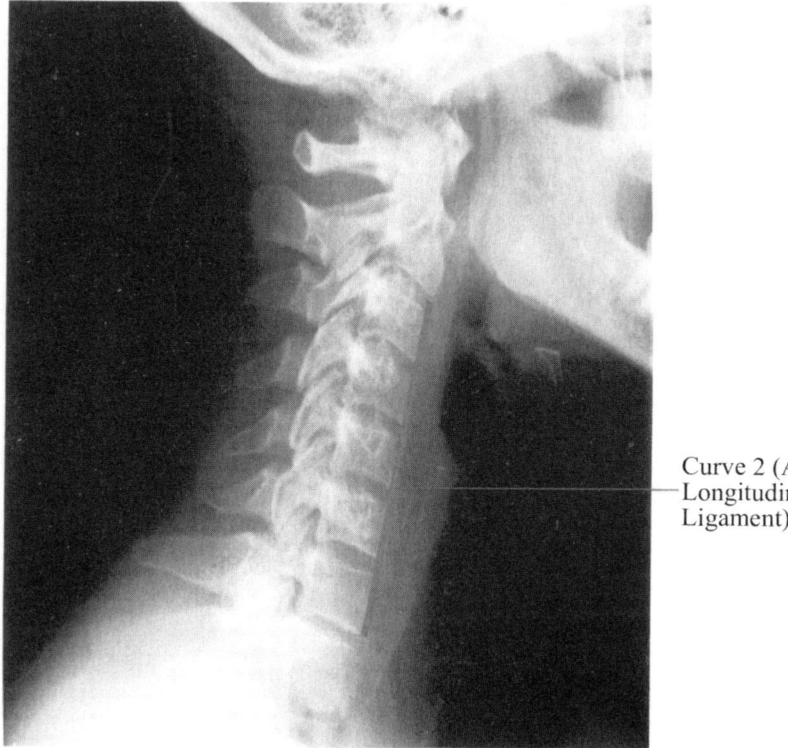

*Figure 2.19   Curve 2 (anterior vertebral body line or anterior
longitudinal ligament line).*

angulation between adjacent vertebrae of more than 11 degrees is suggestive
of ligamentous disruption or vertebral dislocation (Galli 1989) (Figure 2.23)
(a 30 degree angle is illustrated).

The line labeled "Curve 4," the posterior facet line, "joins" the posterior
margin of the facets (Figure 2.24). A disruption in this line may be indicative
of facet displacement (Figure 2.25).

The line labeled "Curve 5," the spinolaminal line, joins the anterior margins
of the junctions of the lamina and spinous processes (Figure 2.26).   The
spinolaminal line, in conjunction with the posterior facet line (Curve 4), helps
to assess the laminar-facet distance. An abrupt variation in this distance may
indicate spinal rotation, such as may be associated with unilateral facet dislocation (Young 1992) (Figure 2.27).

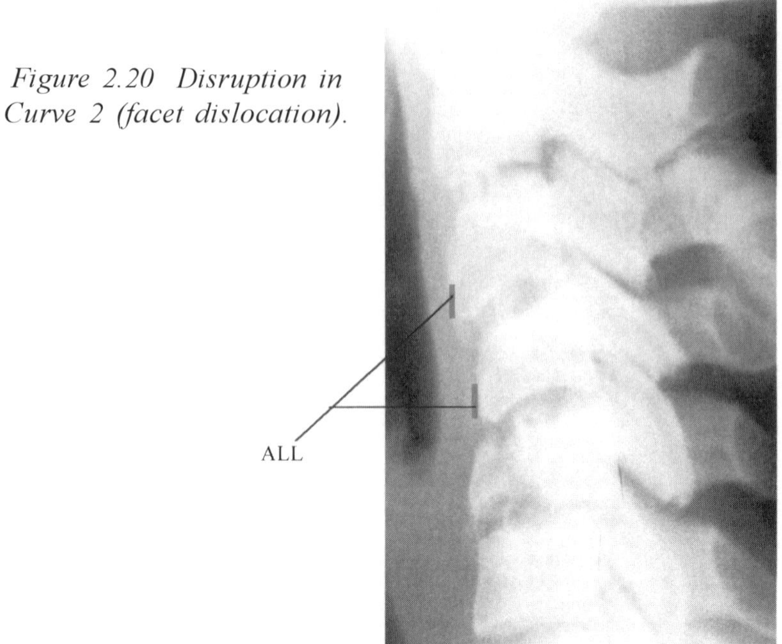

Figure 2.20 Disruption in Curve 2 (facet dislocation).

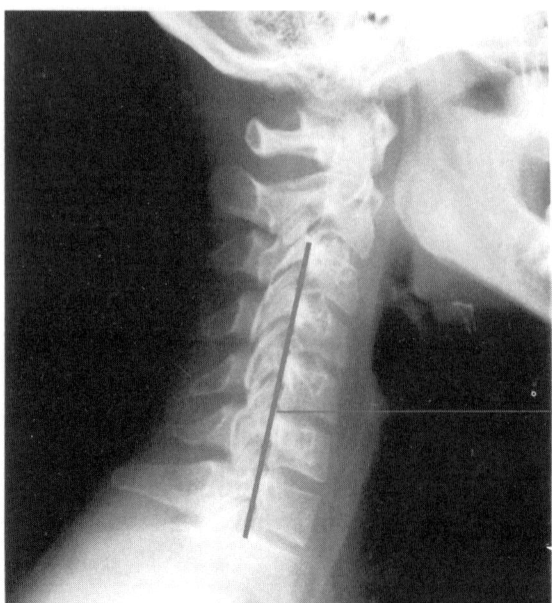

Figure 2.21 Lateral view—Curve 3 (posterior vertebral body line) (posterior longitudinal ligament line).

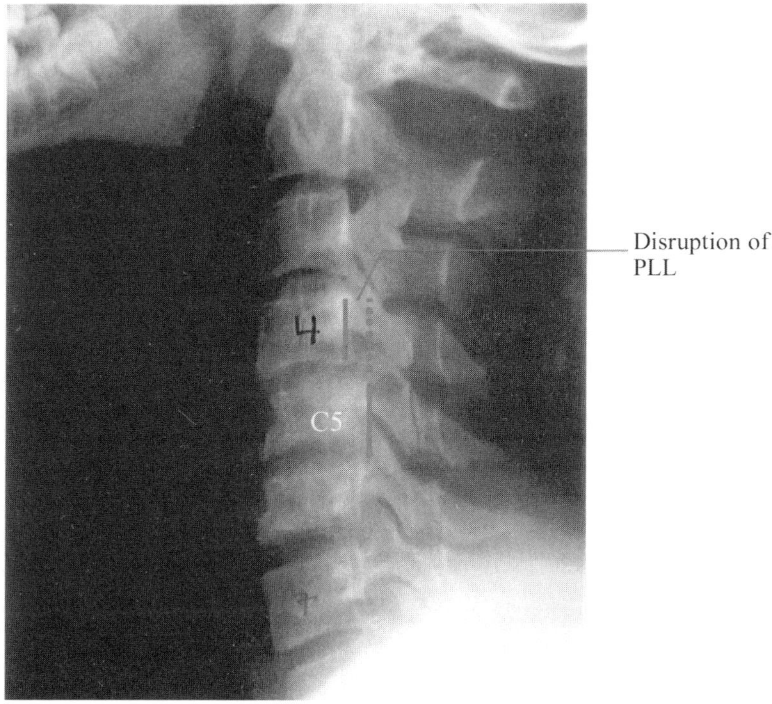

*Figure 2.22 Disruption of Curve 3 (posterior vertebral body line)
and posterior longitudinal ligament.*

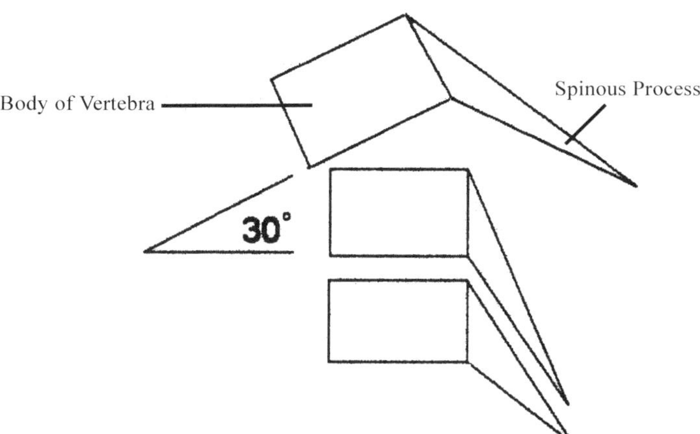

Figure 2.23 Angulation between adjacent vertebrae.

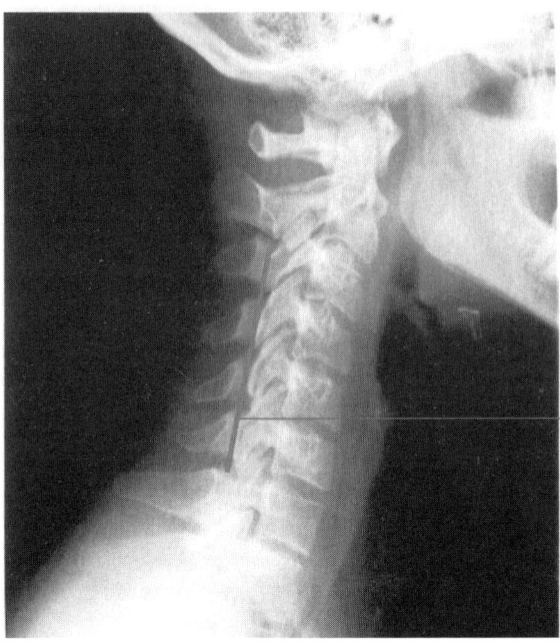

Figure 2.24 Curve 4— Posterior facet line.

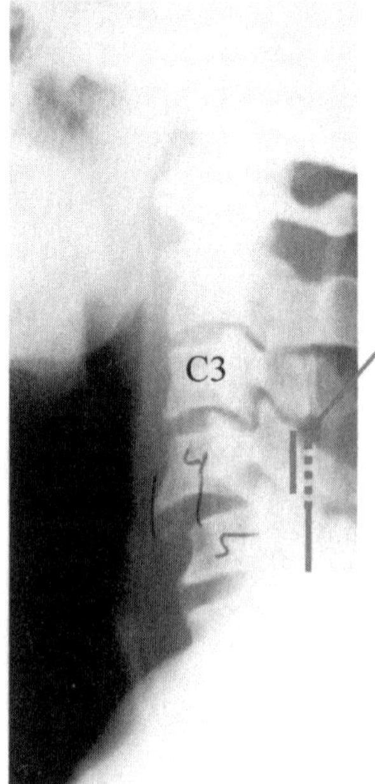

Figure 2.25 Lateral view— disruption in Curve 4 (facet dislocation).

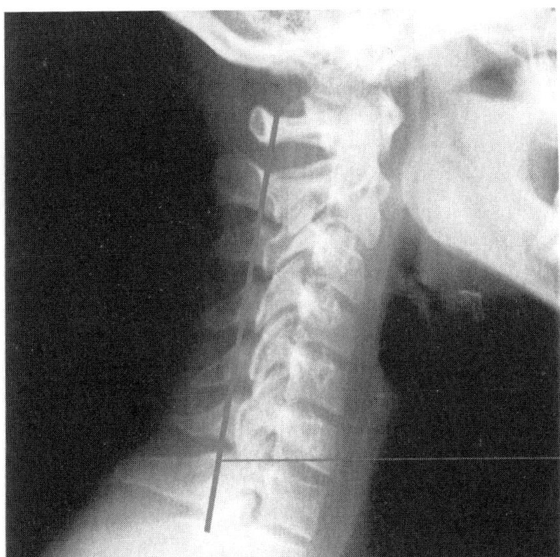

Figure 2.26 Lateral view—Curve 5 (spinolaminal line).

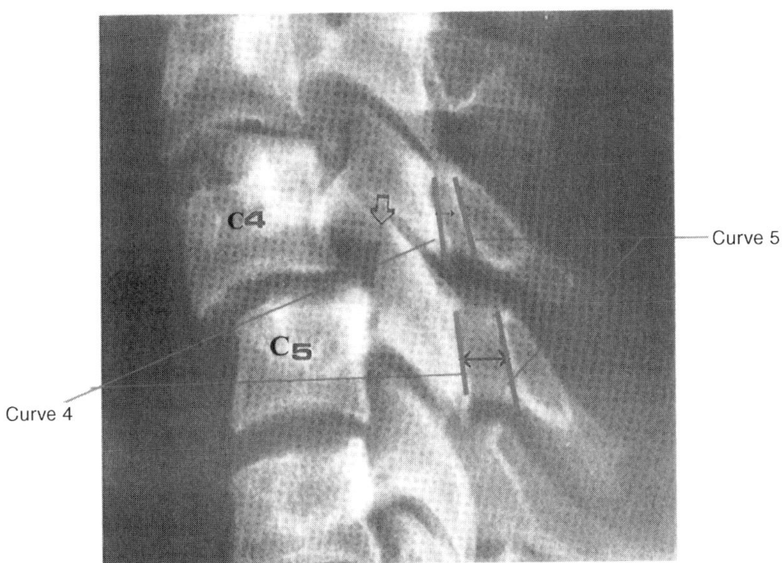

Figure 2.27 Unilateral facet dislocation (as indicated by Curves 4 and 5). [Reproduced with permission. Source: Harris, J.; Mirvis, S. Radiology of Acute Cervical Spine Trauma, *3rd Edition. Williams & Wilkins (Baltimore), 1996.]*

Curves 3 and 5 approximate the anterior and posterior boundaries, respectively, of the spinal canal. Although it might seem that a decrease in the distance between these two curves at any level would indicate a compromise of the canal, this may not be the case. Quite the contrary, the canal is wider at the upper cervical spine than at the lower cervical spine. However, if the A-P distance is less than the diameter of the spinal cord (10–13 mm) at any point, it raises the possibility that a bony structure is impinging on the spinal cord (Figure 2.28) (Galli 1989).[15]

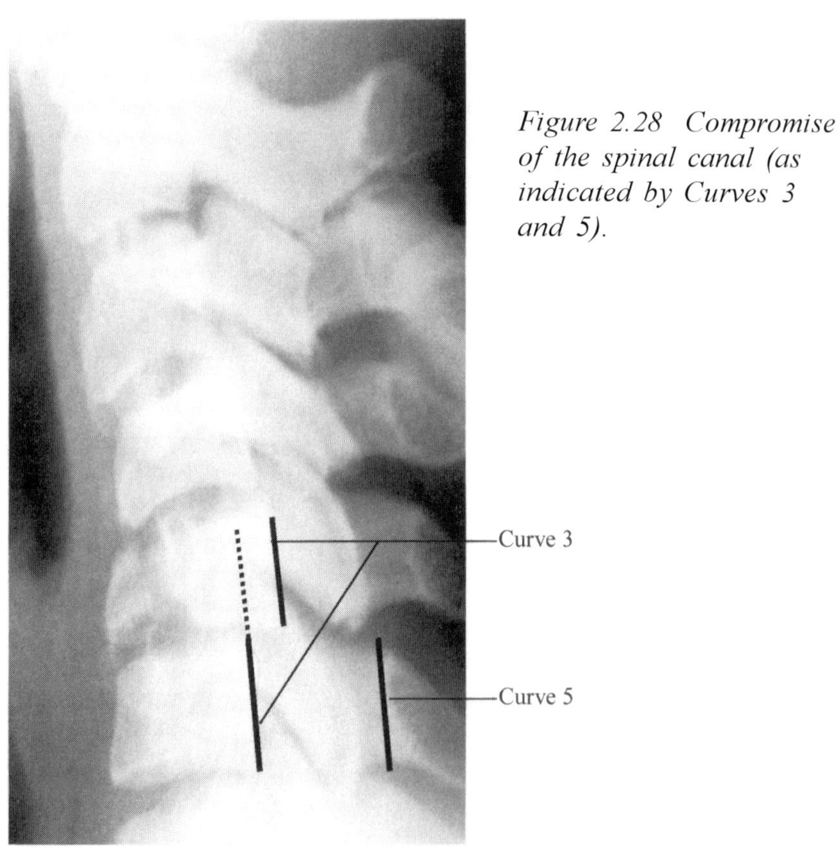

Figure 2.28 Compromise of the spinal canal (as indicated by Curves 3 and 5).

---

[15] Note that the 10–13 mm rule should be applied only to a "true" lateral projection, i.e., one in which the mid-sagittal plane is parallel to the plane of the film. (As will be discussed later, the trueness of a lateral projection can be assessed using Curve 5.)

The spinolaminal line (Curve 5) also provides useful information regarding the orientation of the x-ray. If it is a "true" lateral view, the left and right articular masses will be superimposed on each other, and this will show as a single line (Figure 2.29). If the subject's head is slightly rotated at the time of imaging, the masses will not appear superimposed, but will appear as a tapering pair of lines. If the entire body is rotated, the masses again will not appear superimposed, but will appear as a series of parallel double lines (Galli 1989) (Figure 2.30). If the radiograph is not a true lateral view (as is often the case under emergency room conditions), the alignment of each group of facet joints may be examined separately, and closer scrutiny may be afforded to the frontal and/or oblique views.

The line labeled "Curve 6," the spinous process tip line (Figure 2.31), may be somewhat less smooth than the other four lines because of the great variation in the amount of posterior projection of the processes of the different vertebrae. However, a marked discontinuity may be indicative of injury, such as a spinous process fracture or bilateral facet fracture (Figure 2.32).

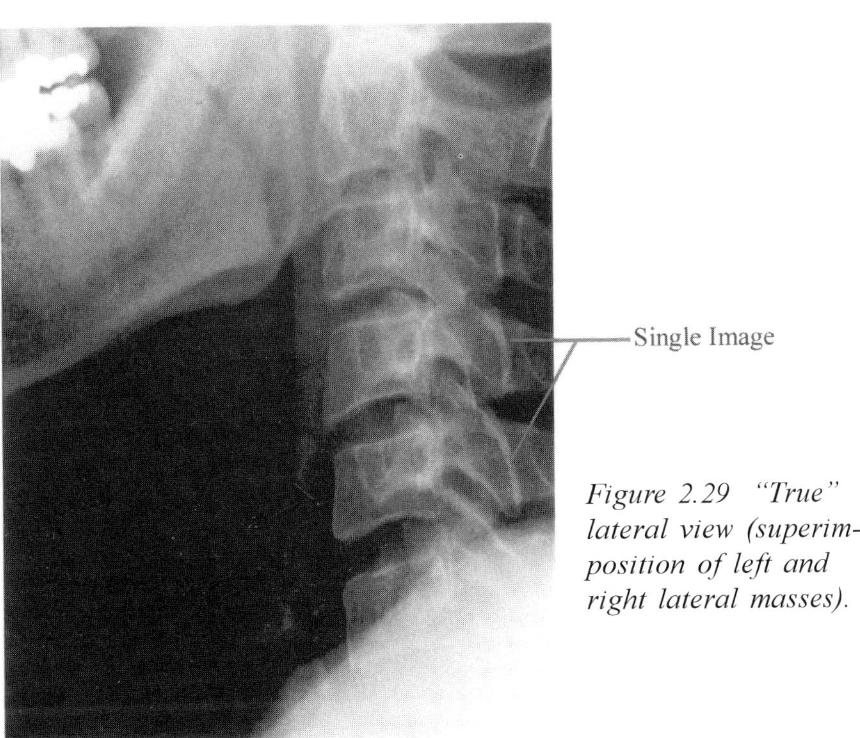

Figure 2.29 "True" lateral view (superimposition of left and right lateral masses).

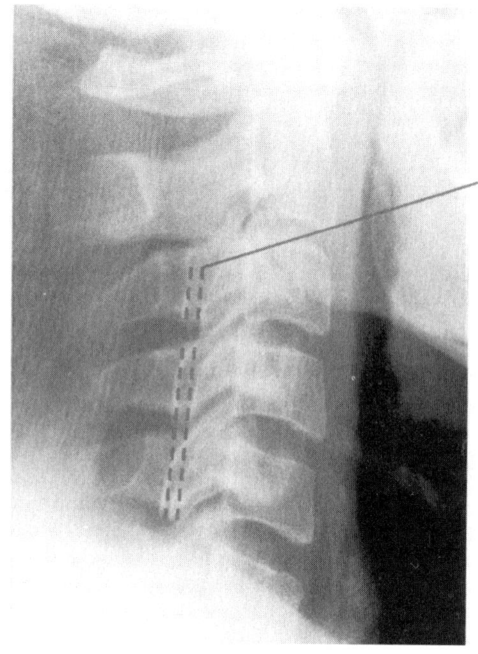

Figure 2.30 Effect of rotation on appearance of spinolaminal line (Curve 4).

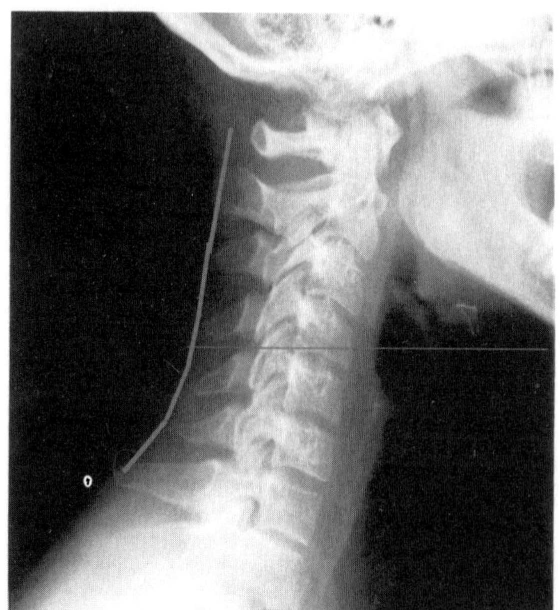

Figure 2.31 Lateral view— Curve 6 (spinous process tip line).

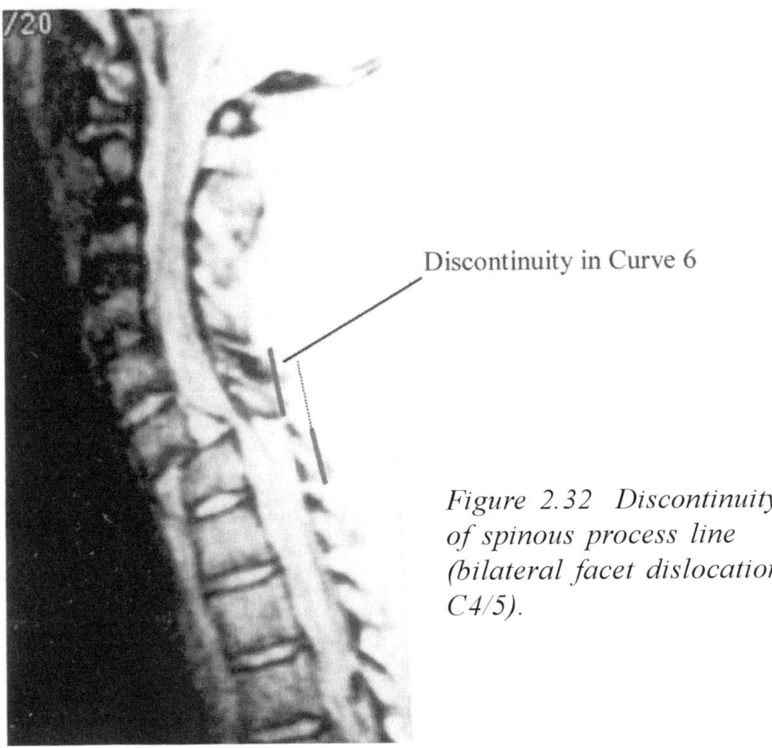

Figure 2.32 Discontinuity of spinous process line (bilateral facet dislocation, C4/5).

The height of each vertebral body should be rather constant in lateral view. For a given vertebra, even a small variation in height (3 mm) is consistent with a compressive fracture of the vertebra (Galli 1989).

Cartilage

The "C" of the "ABC'S" mnemonic stands for cartilage, which refers to the intervertebral disc. Spacing between two adjacent vertebrae should be constant. If this spacing is wider anteriorly, it may be indicative of an extension-type injury. If this space is wider posteriorly (also referred to as "fanning" of the vertebral processes), it may be indicative of a flexion-type injury (discussed in Chapter 3). Note that "normal" intervertebral spacing tends to be greater between adjacent lower cervical vertebrae than between adjacent upper cervical vertebrae, i.e., the discs of the lower cervical vertebrae are thicker than the discs of the upper cervical vertebrae, in the superior-inferior dimension.

Soft Tissue Swelling

Additional information, beyond that provided by the "alignment curves," may sometimes be obtained by an examination of the soft tissue region between the anterior of the vertebrae and the posterior of the pharynx—the pre-vertebral (or retro-pharyngeal) soft tissue. This region is shown as the area between Curves 1 and 2, in Figure 2.18. Although in general, pre-vertebral soft tissue swelling may reflect a number of different conditions, in the trauma setting it most often will indicate bleeding and the resultant accumulation of blood (Galli 1989), which in turn is caused by ligamentous rupture and/or bone fracture.

Pre-vertebral swelling may be the only indicator of injury on the plain film lateral radiograph. Unfortunately, the absence or presence of pre-vertebral soft tissue swelling can be difficult to assess. Generally, pre-trauma radiographs are not available for comparison; thus, the amount of pre-vertebral soft tissue swelling (post-trauma) must be compared to what is typical for the population, rather than what was "normal" for the particular individual. Unfortunately, the depth of "normal" pre-vertebral soft tissue varies considerably (Penning 1989), and only for relatively large values of soft tissue measurement does it become a reliable indicator of the presence of swelling (and presumably, of trauma) (Young 1992).

Pre-vertebral swelling may appear on an image without associated injury (e.g., from swallowing). Conversely, injury may occur without pre-vertebral swelling (e.g., the blood may accumulate remote from the pre-vertebral region). As a rule of thumb, the distance between C3 and the air column of the trachea should not exceed 2/3 of the diameter of the body of C3 (Straub 1989). More precisely, soft tissue measurements in excess of 7 mm (at C3 level) tend to indicate some likelihood of underlying injury, and measurements in excess of 10 mm are frequently associated with related injury (Young 1992).

Anterior-Posterior View

As discussed previously, the term "anterior-posterior (A-P) view" indicates that the x-ray source is located in front of the neck, the x-ray beam travels through the neck front-to-back, and the film to be exposed is positioned behind the neck (Figure 2.33). This arrangement means that the back of the neck is closer to the film than is the front of the neck, and therefore posterior surfaces will be emphasized in the A-P radiographic view.

An A-P view is frequently used to supplement a lateral view. As such, it provides additional information regarding the spinous process, the pillars, and the uncovertebral joints (Figures 2.33 and 2.34). This information primarily

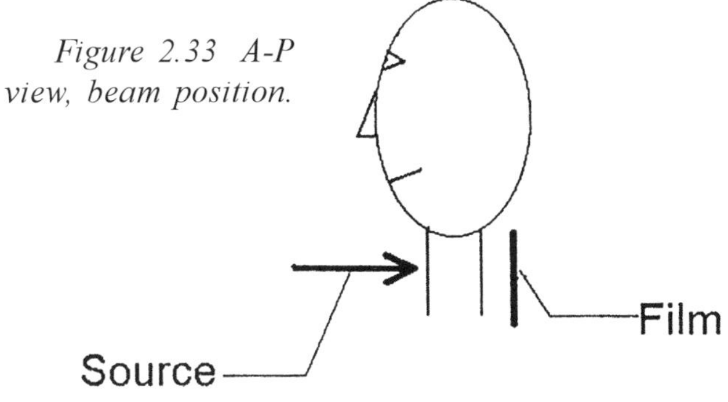

Figure 2.33   A-P view, beam position.

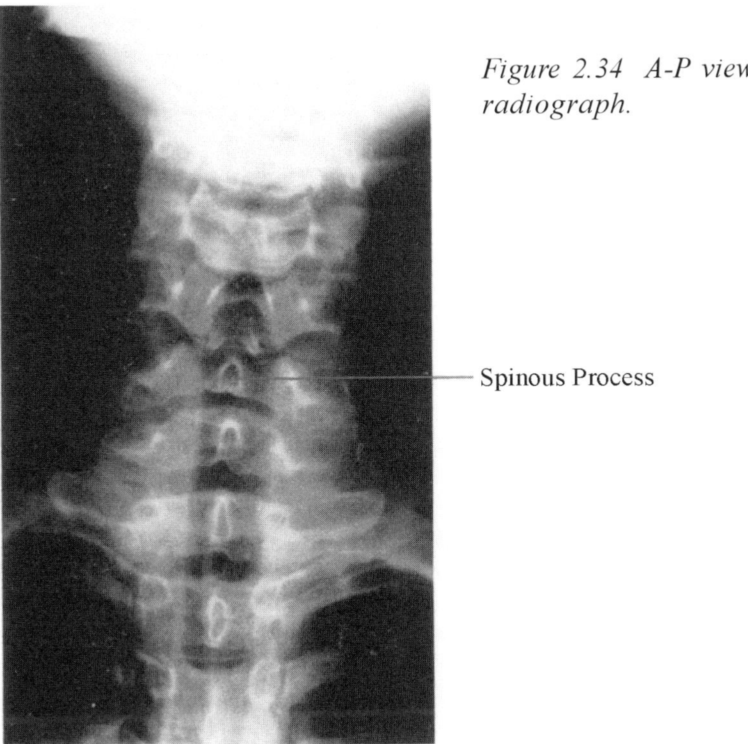

Figure 2.34   A-P view, radiograph.

helps to assess the lateral masses (pillars), especially facet dislocations or lateral mass fracture. The AP view in Figure 2.35 shows damage to both the right and left facet joints and a rotation of one of the affected vertebra, as indicated by the C5 spinous process being displaced from midline (Figure 2.35).

There should be good alignment (straight line or smooth curve) of the spinous processes and the pedicles. Any indication to the contrary may indicate spinal rotation, such as that characteristic of unilateral facet fracture/dislocation.

The lateral margins of the pillars should present as smooth, gradual curves. Abrupt changes or discontinuities in the lateral margin "curve" may indicate facet fracture and/or dislocation. Because the trachea or windpipe is normally filled with air and air transmits relatively high levels of x-rays to the film, the trachea appears in radiographs as a dark column-like structure (Figure 2.36) and may be referred to as the "tracheal air column." After injury, blood accumulation and/or tissue swelling may occur next to the trachea and thereby displace or deform it. For this reason, if the trachea does not appear centered and

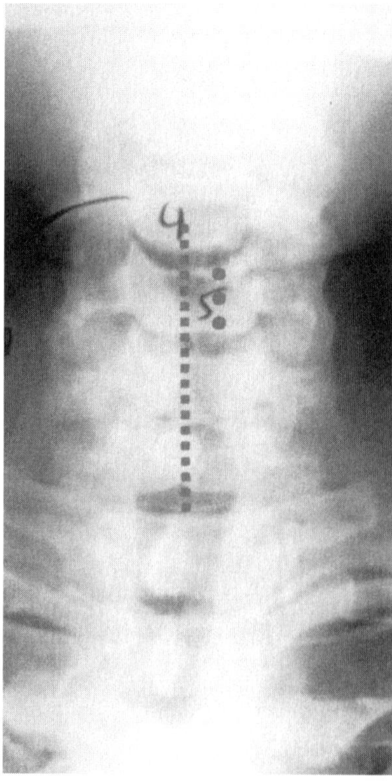

Figure 2.35 A-P view, displacement of spinous process from midline (radiograph).

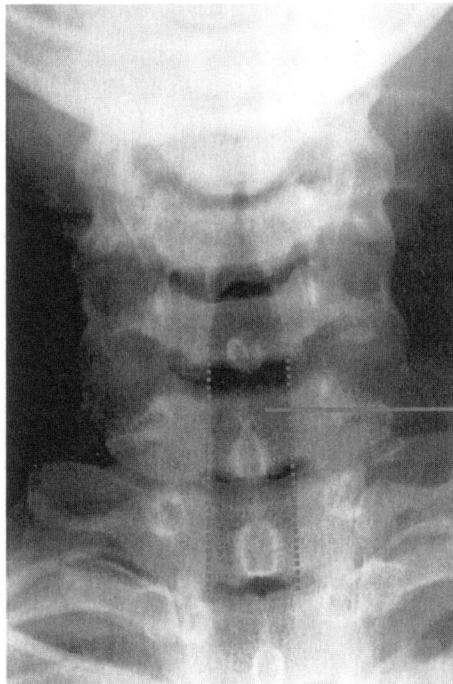

*Figure 2.36
Tracheal air
column
(A-P view).*

symmetrical, especially at the vocal cord level (Rhea 1988), it may indicate trauma—not usually to the trachea per se, but rather to the cervical spine.

The uncovertebral joints (sometimes called the joints of Luschka) (Figure 1.12), consist of the articulating lateral edges of bodies of adjacent vertebrae. The elevated edge of the body of the lower vertebra is called the uncinate process, hence uncovertebral (discussed in Chapter 1). These joints should be symmetrical and vertically oriented.

Odontoid View

The odontoid view, as its name implies, is used for viewing the odontoid process (dens) of C2 and other structures of the upper cervical spine. The mandible on a "regular" A-P view typically obscures the upper cervical spine region, and thus the odontoid view serves as an A-P (anterior-posterior) view of the upper cervical spine. To "eliminate" the mandible, the odontoid view is usually A-P in orientation, but with the x-ray beam aimed at the mouth (Figure 2.37).

The purpose of this positioning is to produce an image with the mandible, teeth, and occiput essentially removed, i.e., not superimposed on the odontoid (Figures 2.38). The resulting image can provide much information regarding bone fracture and/or ligament disruption. More specifically, the odontoid view is used to check for fracture of either the dens (Figure 2.39) or of the ring of C1 and for ligamentous injury, as evidenced by the improper alignment between C1 and C2.

The lateral displacement of both halves of C1 is indicative of ligamentous and/or bony injury (Figure 2.40). Fracture of the bony ring of C1 may also be

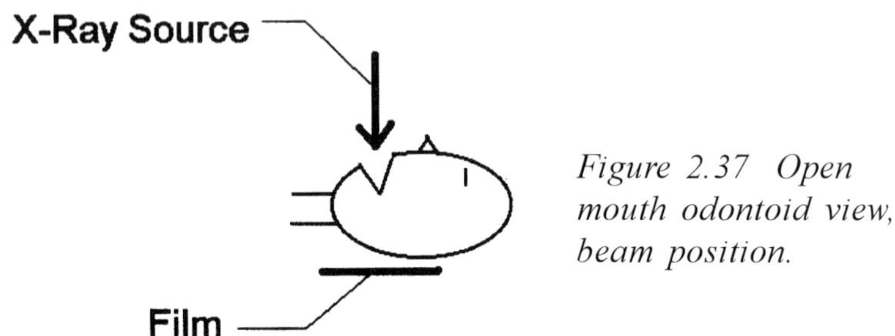

Figure 2.37 Open mouth odontoid view, beam position.

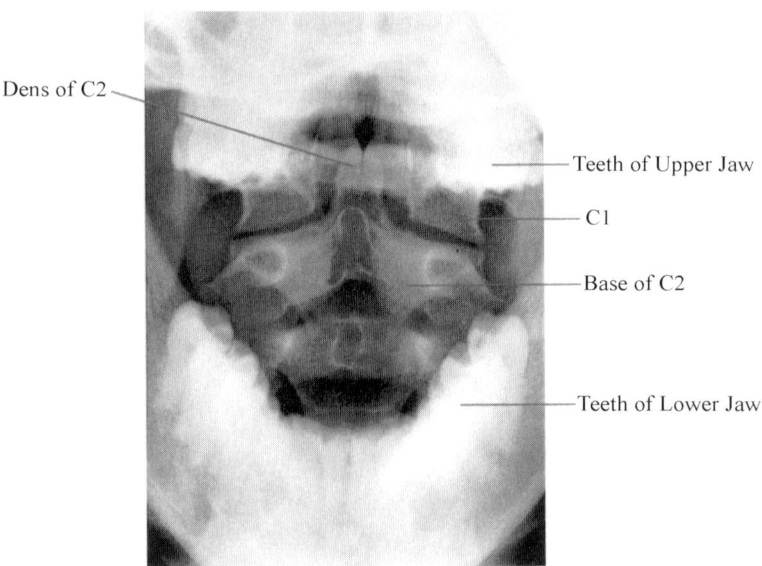

Figure 2.38 Open mouth odontoid view, radiograph.

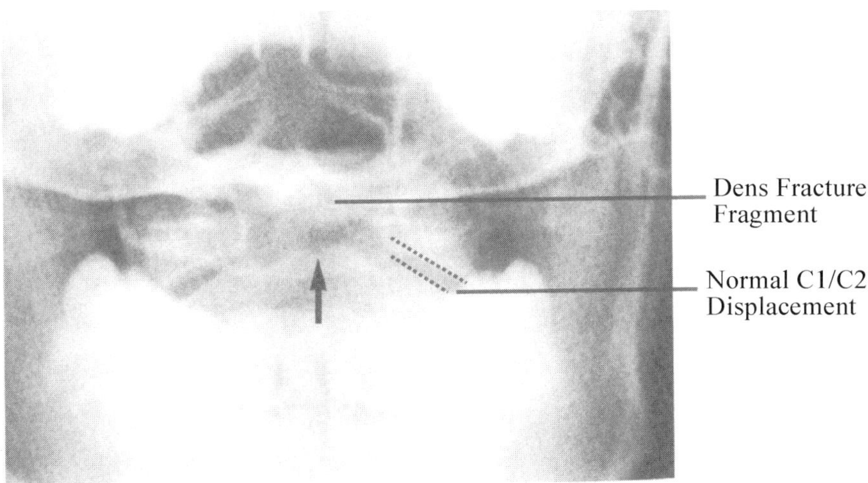

*Figure 2.39   Open mouth odontoid view, C2 fracture (of dens).
[Reproduced with permission.   Source: Camins, M.B.; O'Leary, P.F.*
Disorders of the Cervical Spine. *Williams & Wilkins (Baltimore), 1992.]*

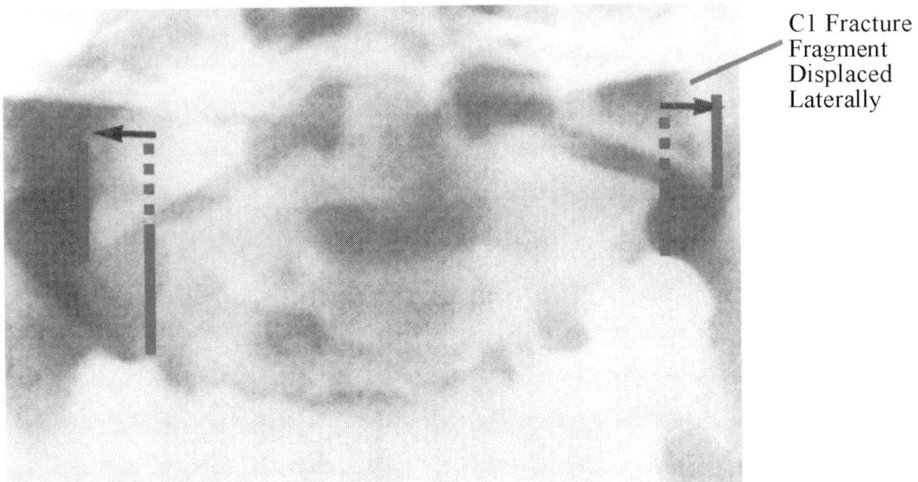

*Figure 2.40   Open mouth odontoid view (Jefferson fracture [C1]).
[Reproduced with permission.   Source: Camins, M.B.; O'Leary, P.F.*
Disorders of the Cervical Spine. *Williams & Wilkins (Baltimore), 1992.]*

observed with CT (Figure 2.41). A bilateral fracture involving both anterior and posterior elements of C2 is often referred to as a Jefferson fracture. It should be noted that displacement of both halves (lateral masses) of C1 to the same side (either right or left) of the dens is not indicative of injury (Figure 2.42).

Although the odontoid region is usually imaged with the mouth open (the "open mouth" view), the odontoid region may also be imaged with the mouth closed. This "closed mouth odontoid" view may be necessary if there is concern that the head and neck movement required to obtain proper positioning for the open mouth view may exacerbate an existing injury. The closed mouth odontoid view is oriented to have the odontoid superimposed on the image of the foramen magnum, the large opening in the base of the skull. This, in turn, provides a plain black background on the image and permits easy viewing of the odontoid region. This closed mouth odontoid view is sometimes referred to as the Fuchs view (Figure 2.43). In the remainder of this text, unless otherwise noted, odontoid view will refer to open mouth odontoid.

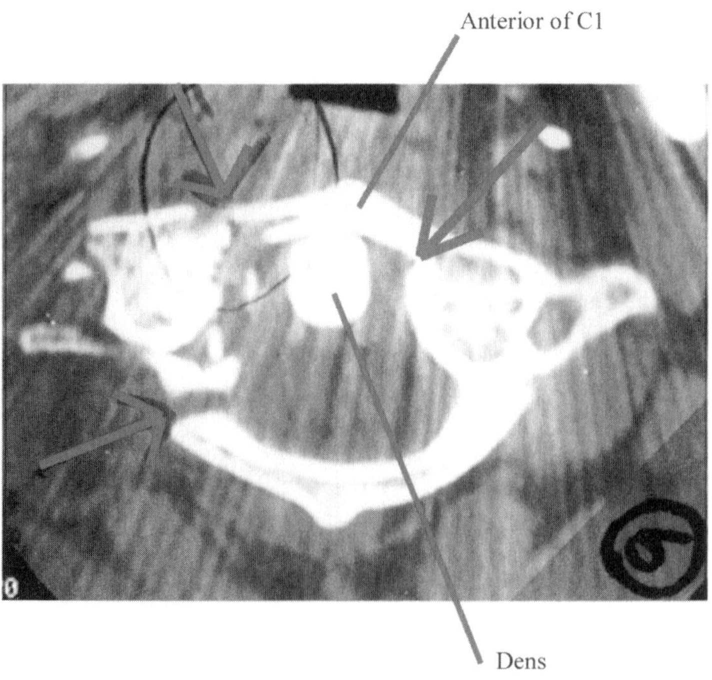

Figure 2.41 Jefferson fracture (C1), CT (axial view).

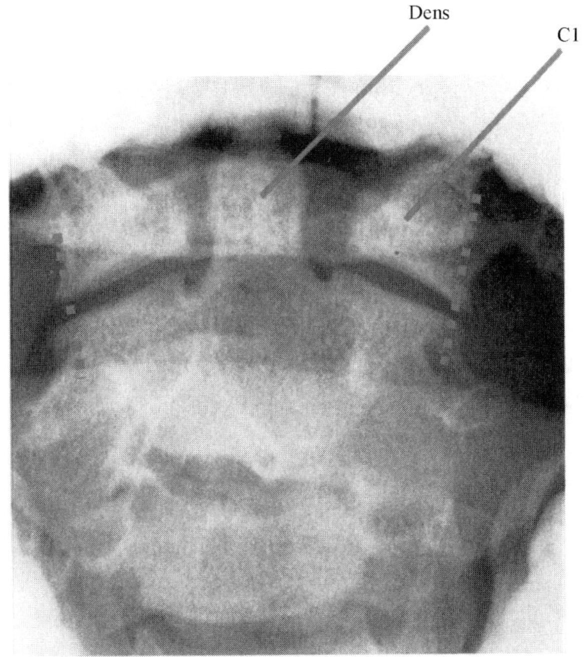

Figure 2.42 C1 lateral mass displacement without injury (normal).

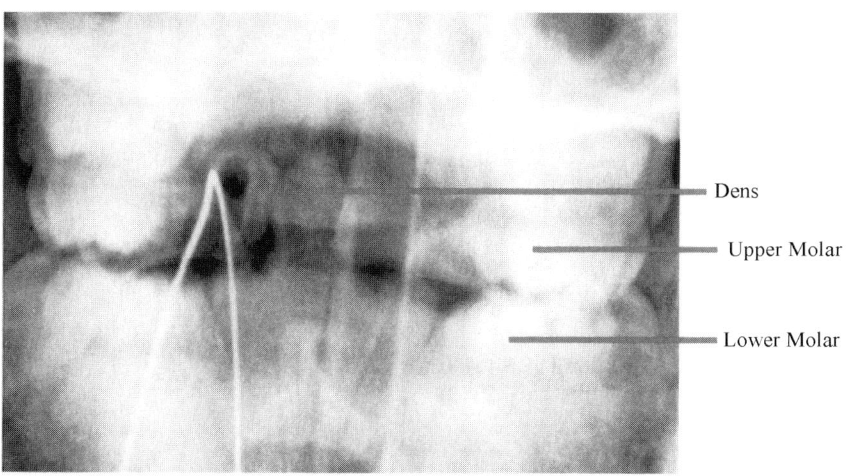

Figure 2.43 Closed mouth odontoid view (Fuch's view).

Occasionally, there may appear to be a fracture in the radiograph, even though no fracture has occurred. An example is when the radiograph seemingly shows a fracture at the base of the dens, but the "fracture line" is actually an artifact of the imaging process, namely, it is due to the superimposed inferior aspect of the C1 ring (and is referred to as the Mach band or Mach effect). A similar effect can occur if the image of an upper incisor is superimposed on the image of the odontoid (Huebner 1994). A third possibility is that a non-union of the C1 arch (Figure 2.44, bottom) will appear to be a dens fracture (Figure 2.44, top).

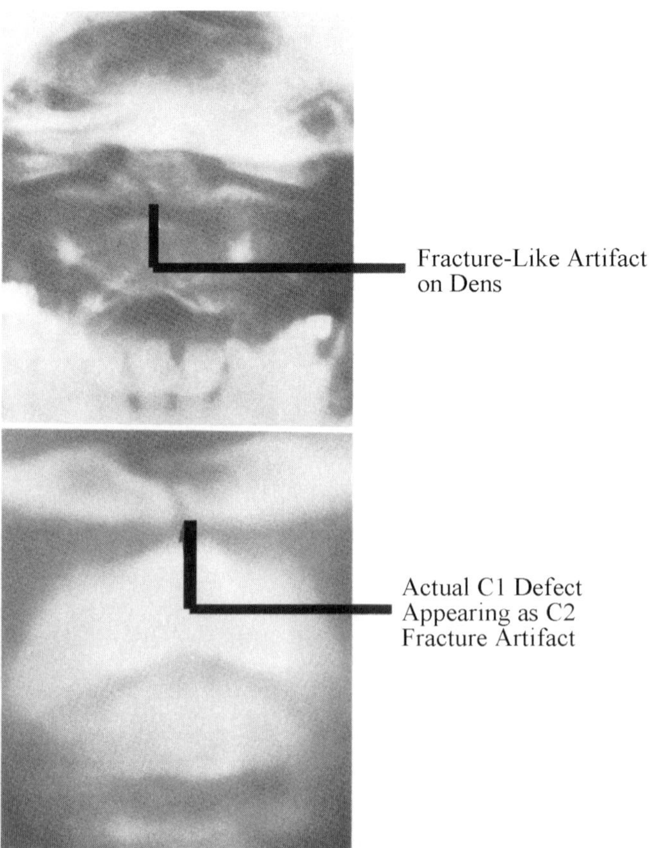

*Figure 2.44   Open mouth odontoid view, fracture-like artifact.
[Reproduced with permission.   Source: Camins, M.B.; O'Leary, P.F.
Disorders of the Cervical Spine.   Williams & Wilkins (Baltimore), 1992.]*

Oblique Views (Left and Right)

The oblique view (Figure 2.45) permits evaluation of the pedicles, lamina and facets, and the openings of the neural foramina. Perhaps the most telltale sign in this view involves the laminae. These should have an orderly "shingled" appearance (Figure 2.46), and any disruption of the shingles may be indicative of injury, such as unilateral facet dislocation (Figure 2.47).

The oblique view may also show compression fractures of the lateral masses (Wasenko 1992). Furthermore, any compromise of the neural foramina may be indicative of injury to one or more nerve roots. (The neural foramina may also be compromised by pre-existing degenerative disease, e.g., the growth of osteophytes [bony spurs] [Figure 2.48].)

The oblique view provides somewhat comparable information to a view called the swimmer's view (which will be discussed next). However, compared to the swimmer's view, the oblique view has the added advantage of not requiring additional movement of the subject's head or neck and not having the arm superimposed on the cervical spine image.

Modified CTL (Cross-Table Lateral) View and Swimmer's View

If the lower cervical spine (down to C7/T1) is not adequately displayed on the CTLV, a supplemental view may be used—either the modified CTLV or the swimmer's view. (These alternatives are most often required on heavily muscled or obese individuals.)

The swimmer's view is taken with the subject's contralateral arm raised over his or her head (Figure 2.49), such as when a swimmer is doing the Australian

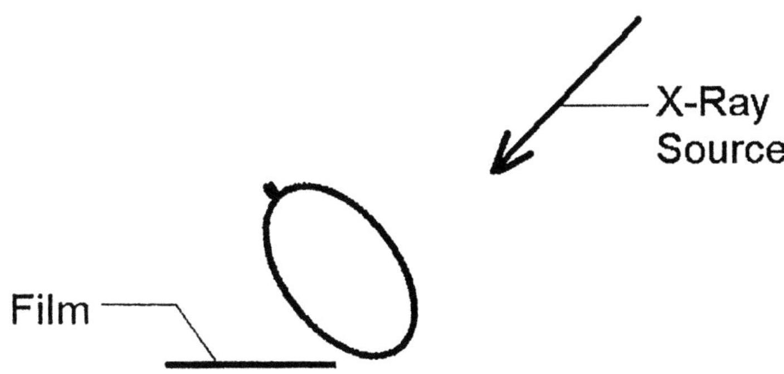

Figure 2.45 Oblique view, beam position.

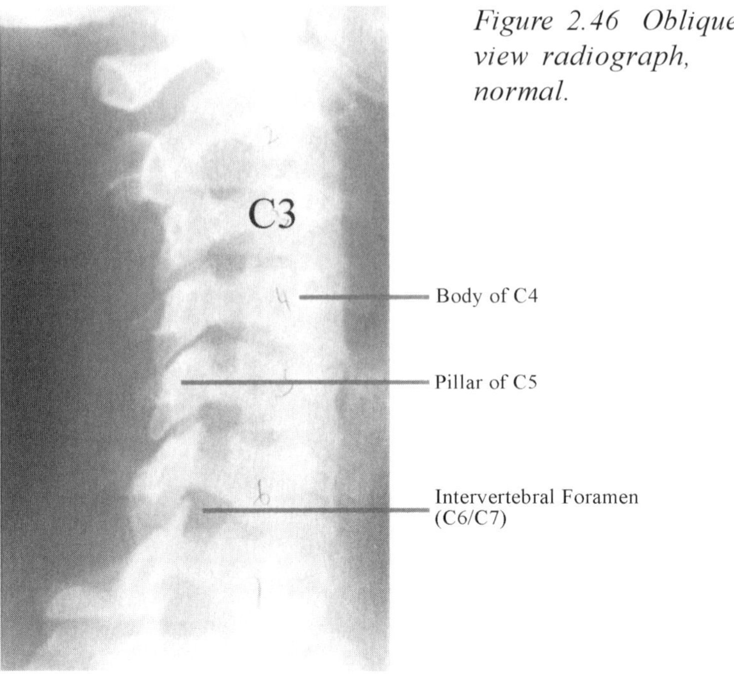

Figure 2.46 Oblique view radiograph, normal.

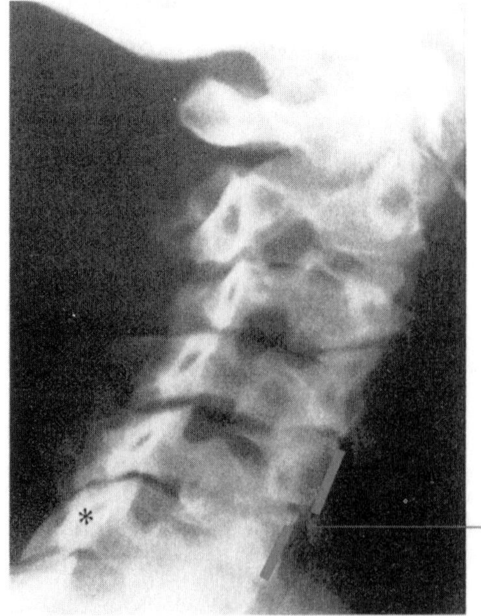

Figure 2.47 Oblique view, radiograph (showing unilateral facet dislocation). [Reproduced with permission. Source: Harris, J.; Harris, W.; Novelline, R. Radiology of Emergency Medicine, *3rd Edition. Williams & Wilkins (Baltimore), 1993.]*

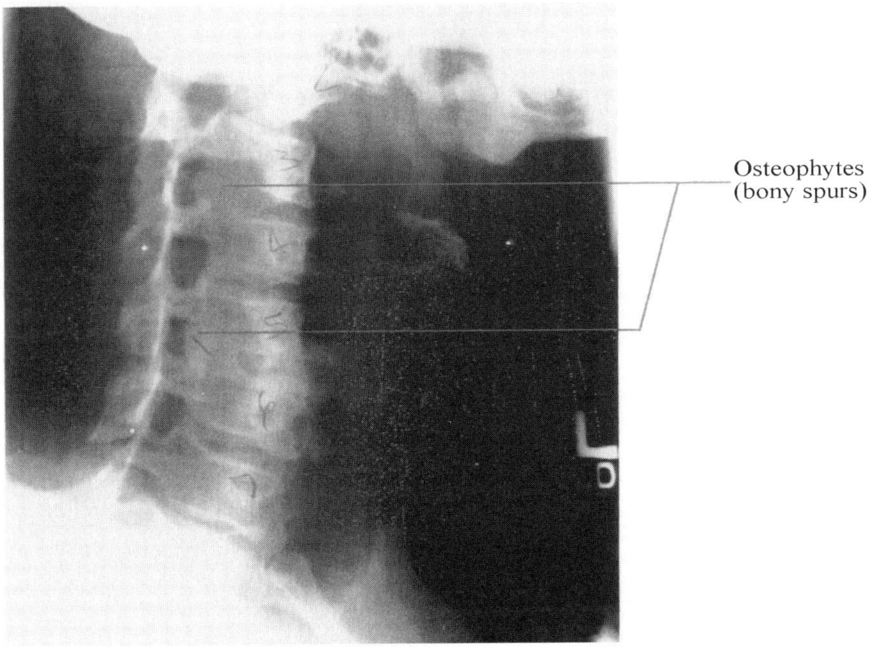

Figure 2.48 Oblique view radiograph (showing degenerative osteophytes [bony spurs] in neural foramen).

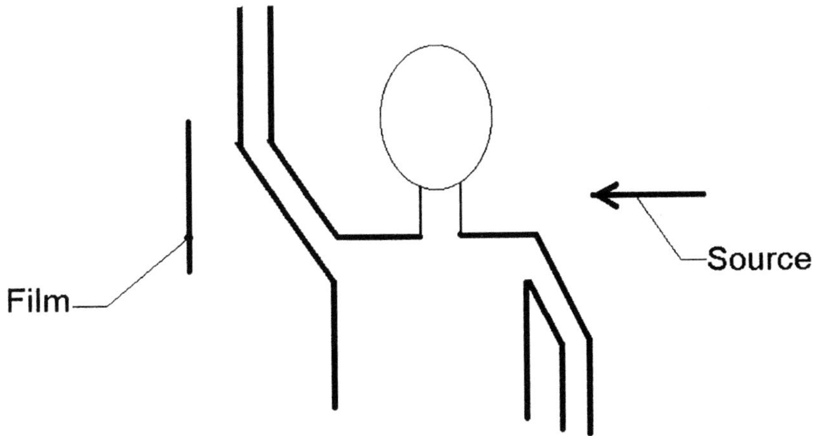

Figure 2.49 Swimmer's view, beam orientation.

crawl stroke. Thus, the shoulder is removed from the picture, thereby providing an image of the lower cervical spine, which does not have an image of the shoulder superimposed on it and is therefore much easier to interpret (Figure 2.50). The need for the swimmer's view is demonstrated by Figure 2.51, which does not show any injury because the shoulder obscures the C6/C7 region of the spine. Figure 2.52, a different lateral image of the same patient, shows the C6/C7 dislocation, which the shoulder had been blocking. (Note that Figure 2.52 is not a swimmer's view but was selected to demonstrate the effect of the shoulder blockage.)

Pillar View

The pillar view is not usually included in the initial, basic set of views but may be added as a supplement. The principal use of the pillar view (Figures 2.53 and 2.54) is to assess pillar fracture, also called articular mass fracture or facet fracture. (Recall that an articular mass may be referred to as a pillar, and the articulating surface of a pillar is often referred to as a facet

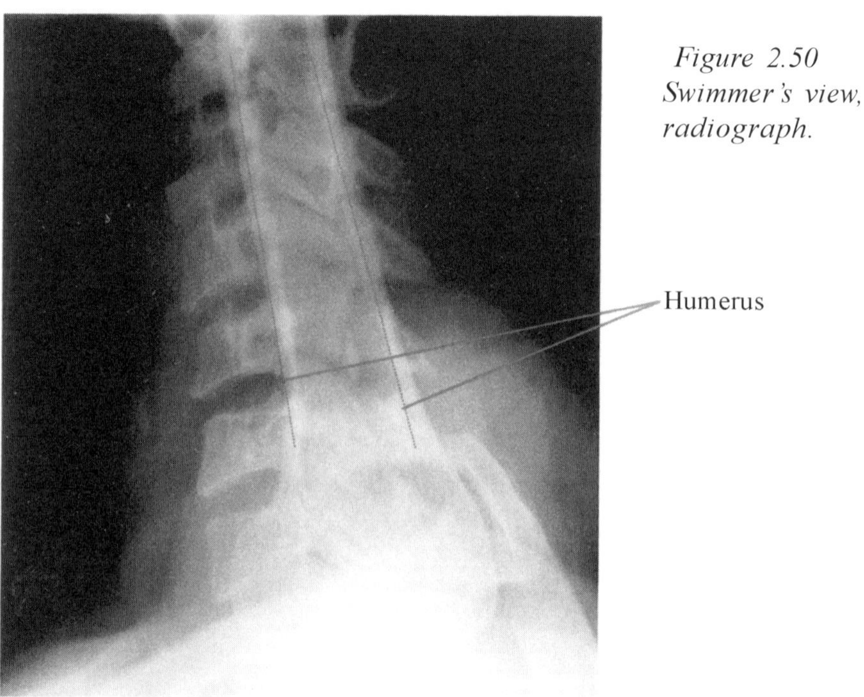

Figure 2.50 Swimmer's view, radiograph.

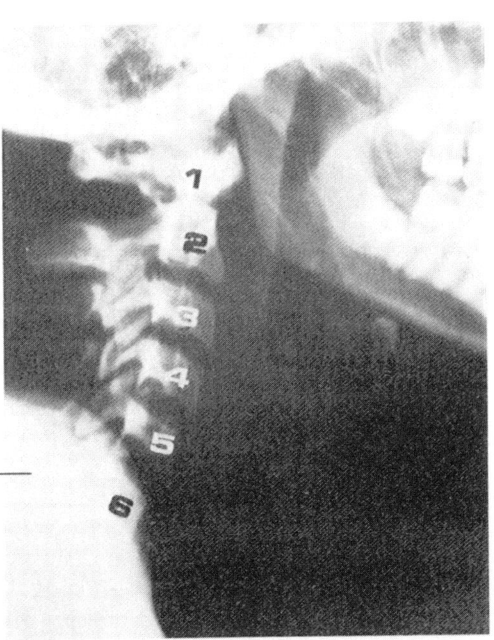

Figure 2.51 Lateral view radiograph (C7 injury blocked by shoulder). [Reproduced with permission. Source: Rockwood, C.A., Jr.; Green, D.P.; Bucholz, R.W. Rockwood and Green's Fractures in Adults, 3rd Edition. Lippincott (Philadelphia), 1991.]

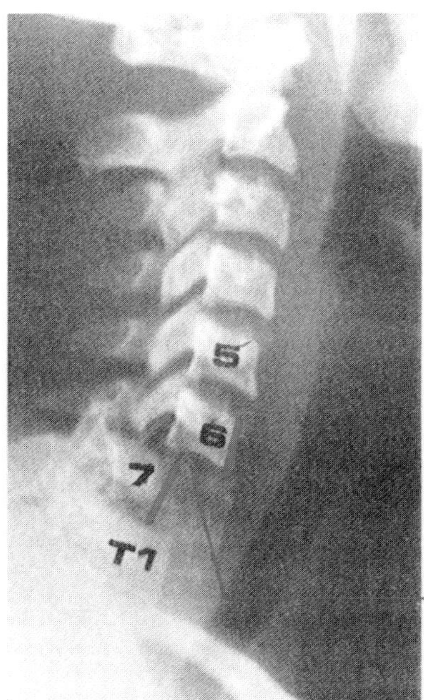

C6/C7 Dislocation

Figure 2.52 Lateral view radiograph showing C6/C7 injury. [Reproduced with permission. Source: Rockwood, C.A., Jr.; Green, D.P.; Bucholz, R.W. Rockwood and Green's Fractures in Adults, 3rd Edition. Lippincott (Philadelphia), 1991.]

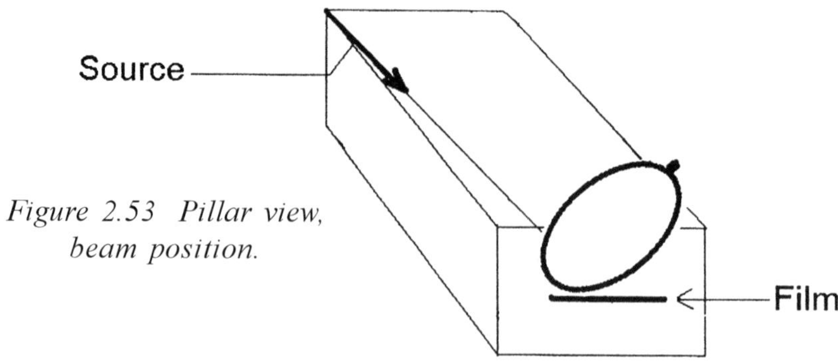

Figure 2.53 Pillar view, beam position.

Figure 2.54 Pillar view, radiograph.

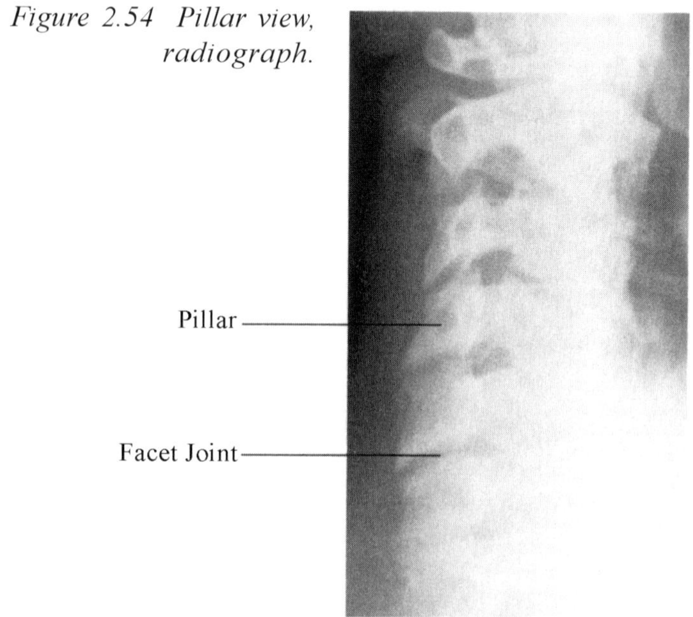

[Chapter 1].) The pillar view is used especially when there is some clinical basis, such as persistent pain or tenderness, for suspecting that a particular injury has occurred (Rhea 1988) but the other views, including oblique, do not confirm the presence of a fracture. Figure 2.55 shows a facet fracture (pillar fracture) as seen on a pillar view. One possible limitation of the pillar view is that it generally requires movement of the patient's head, and such movement may be undesirable.

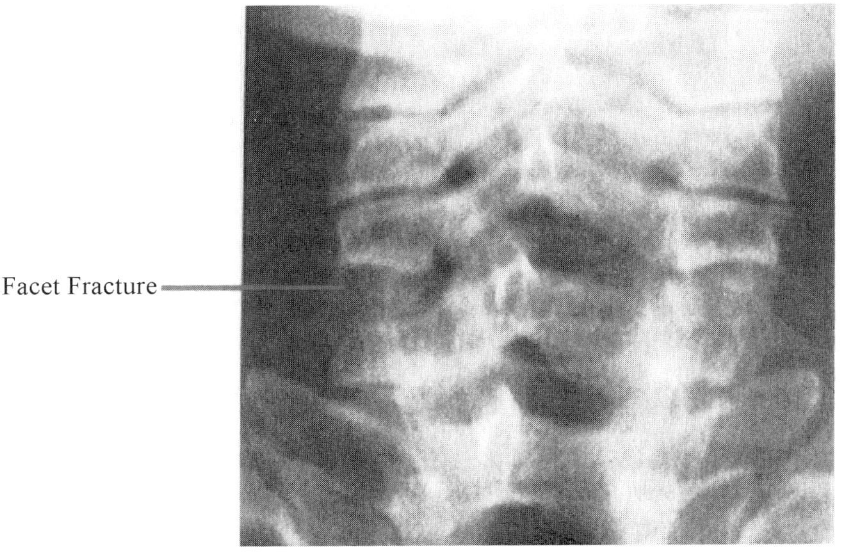

Figure 2.55 Pillar view (showing articular mass [pillar] fracture). [Reproduced with permission. Source: Greenspan, A. Orthopedic Radiology—A Practical Approach, 2nd Edition. Lippincott-Raven (Philadelphia), 1997.]

Flexion View

This view is primarily used to supplement the lateral view to rule out instability of the posterior ligaments. As its name implies, this view is taken with the neck flexed (Figures 2.56 and 2.57). Occasionally, an injury will be more readily observed if the neck is imaged not in the neutral position, but rather is repositioned so that the type of neck movement that caused the injury is recreated. Thus, an injury that was caused by a flexion movement may be better displayed if the neck is flexed.

Figure 2.58, a flexion view, shows a large teardrop fracture fragment and C5/C6 dislocation. To avoid (additional) neurological injury, the movement required to "pose" for this view is performed only after it has been determined that it is all right to flex the neck (i.e., after the C-spine had been "cleared"), and then only when the movement is voluntarily performed by a supervised, cooperative, alert patient (i.e., the patient is not positioned by the radiographic technologist).

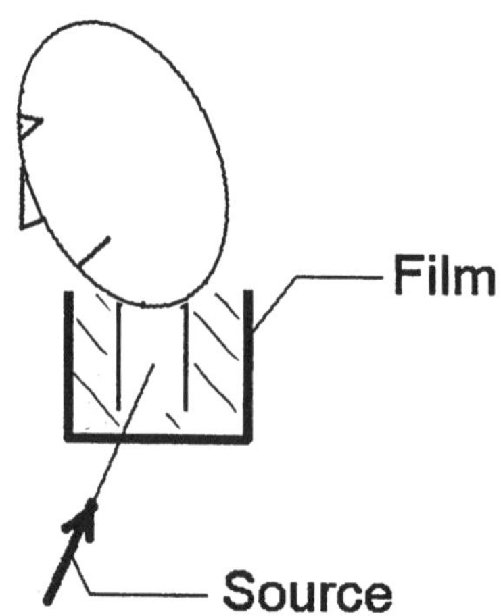

Figure 2.56   Flexion view, position.

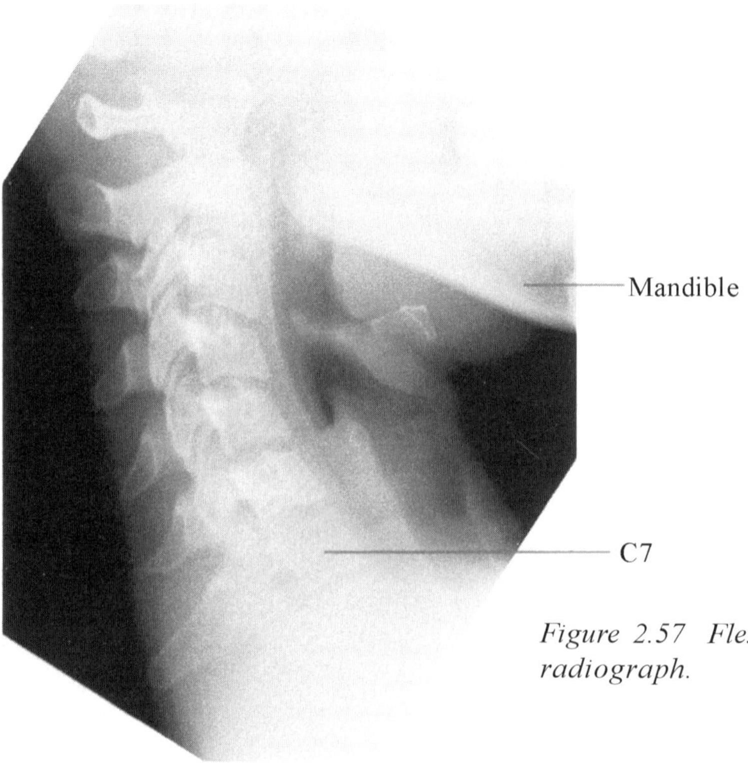

Figure 2.57   Flexion view, radiograph.

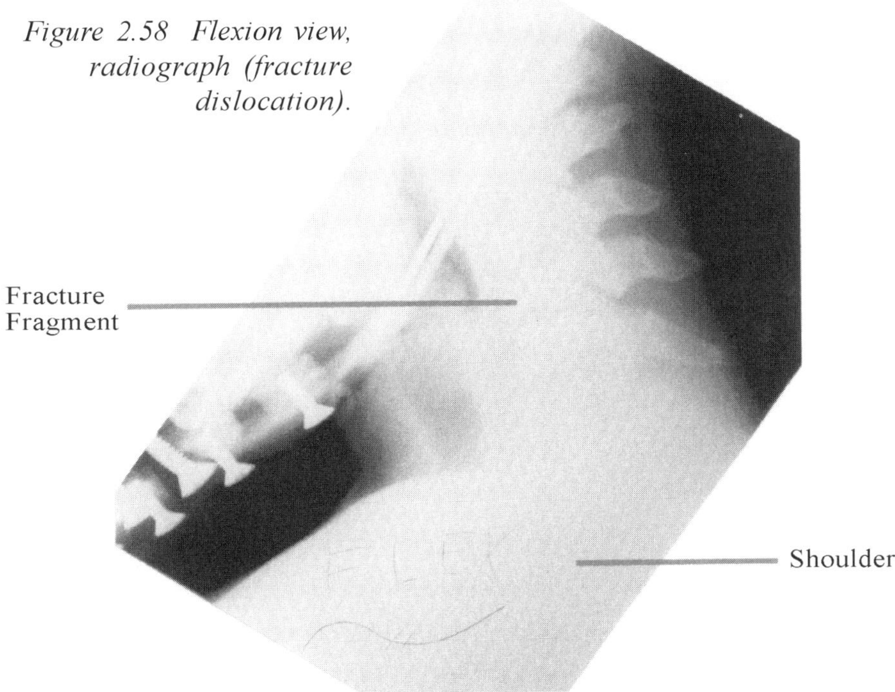

*Figure 2.58   Flexion view,
radiograph (fracture
dislocation).*

Extension View

This view is primarily used to supplement the lateral view to rule out instability of the anterior ligaments. As its name implies, this view is taken with the neck extended (Figures 2.59 and 2.60). To avoid (additional) neurological injury, the movement required to "pose" for this view is performed only after it has been determined that it is all right to extend the neck (i.e., the C-spine had been "cleared"), and then only when the movement is voluntarily performed by a supervised, cooperative, alert patient (i.e., the patient is not positioned by the radiographic technologist). An extension view for the same patient of Figure 2.58 is provided for comparison (Figure 2.61).

Tomograms

The tomogram, mentioned previously, is a relatively recent offshoot of the traditional x-ray. Rather than display the entire depth of a structure, the tomogram

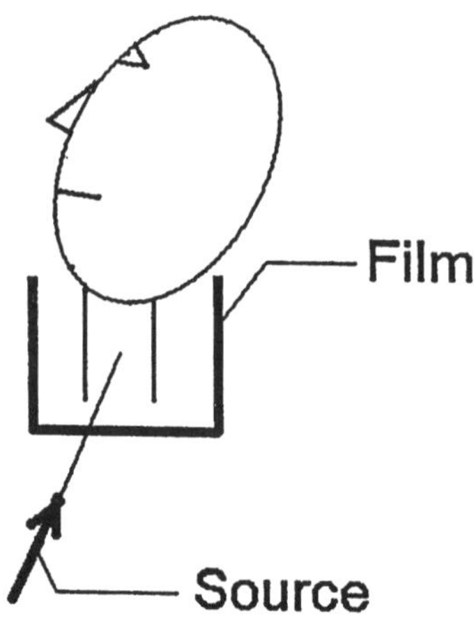

Figure 2.59   Extension view, position.

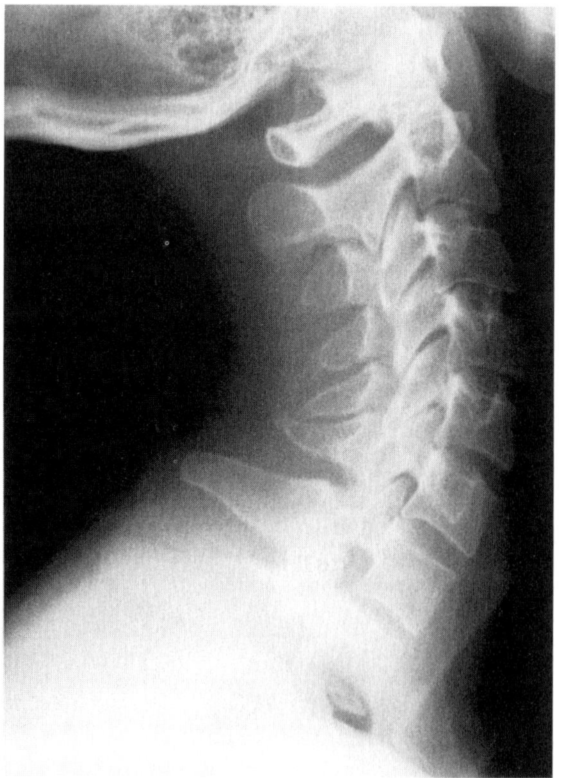

Figure 2.60   Extension view, radiograph.

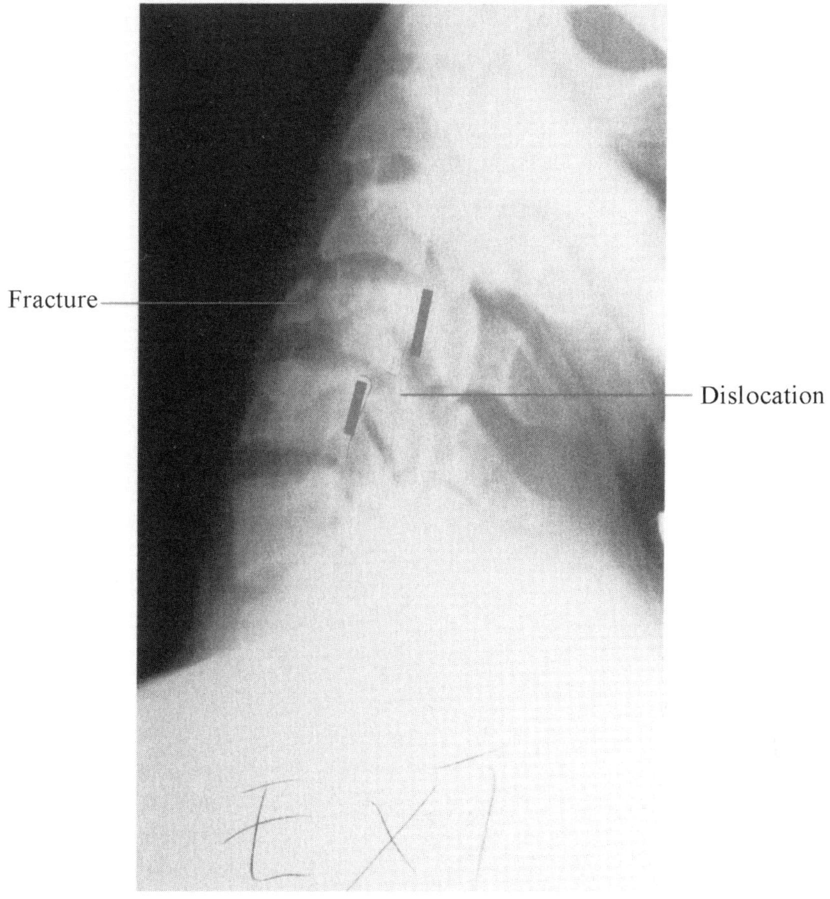

Figure 2.61   Extension view, radiograph (fracture dislocation).

displays a "slice" (somewhat analogous to selecting one slice from a sliced loaf of bread). The tomogram is still a two-dimensional representation of a three-dimensional structure, but tomography enables the operator to select a small region and, in some ways, permits a closer scrutiny of that smaller region. Also, by looking at a series of slices, one can get "the big picture" and an idea of the contribution of each slice or layer to the overall image. One important use of computed tomography (CT) in neck trauma imaging is to detect fracture fragments in the canal or anywhere else near the spinal cord.

Conceptually, a tomogram provides an image that includes only those structures in the plane of interest and excludes structures from all other planes. In practice, structures in other planes are de-emphasized, i.e., blurred, so that it is easier to focus attention on the plane and structure(s) of interest. Tomograms achieve this blurring effect by using a relatively long exposure time (approximately 5 seconds) and by having both the camera and film in motion during the exposure (Figure 2.62). (The patient is not moving.) The movement is precisely controlled such that the film "sees" little or no motion of objects in the focal plane (plane of interest), but the film does see movement and hence produces blurred images of objects in the other planes.

A tomogram can show the location of some fractures that are more difficult to identify in the plain film views. A tomogram loses a lot of the information about structures in other planes, but this loss is characteristic of a single tomogram. A series of tomograms, especially if they are contiguous or better yet, overlapping, can provide much of this additional information (however, these additional images require additional patient exposure to x-rays, imaging time, etc.).

Tomograms may also be generated through the use of computers, in which case the process is referred to as computed tomography or CT. Initially, tomograms were restricted to the axial plane, and this fact was reflected in

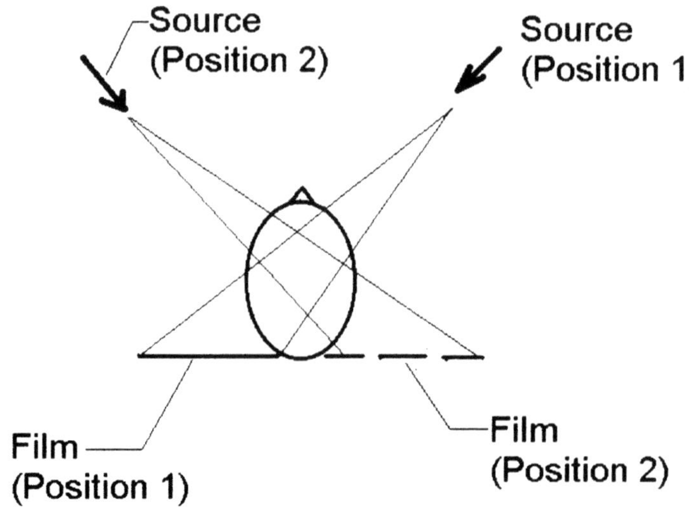

Figure 2.62 Tomogram concept—moving film and camera.

early CT nomenclature—the procedure was referred to as Computed Axial Tomography, or a CAT scan. Today, CT imaging can be in the sagittal or coronal planes as well, but for spinal trauma, CT slices in the transverse (axial) plane (Figure 2.63) are by far the most common. Although the initial spinal imaging is usually in the axial plane, these images may be subsequently reformatted, for example, to provide a sagittal view (Figure 2.64). (Note that, as is typical for reformatted images, the reformatted sagittal view has less definition than the original CT. However, the reformatted image of Figure 2.64 adequately displays a large teardrop fracture of C5 and encroachment of the posterior elements of C5 into the canal and the spinal cord.)

Recent usage tends to lump together axial scans, as well as scans in other planes, under the category of CT. Note that CT may also provide three-dimensional surface contour images (Figure 2.65), and these will be referred to as 3-D CT. Also note that, although CTs use x-rays, CTs will be referred to as "computed tomography" or "CT," without including the term x-ray.

Today, most tomograms are generated with computers, and indeed many imaging facilities have scrapped their conventional tomogram equipment. Some of the reasons why CT has largely replaced conventional tomography are

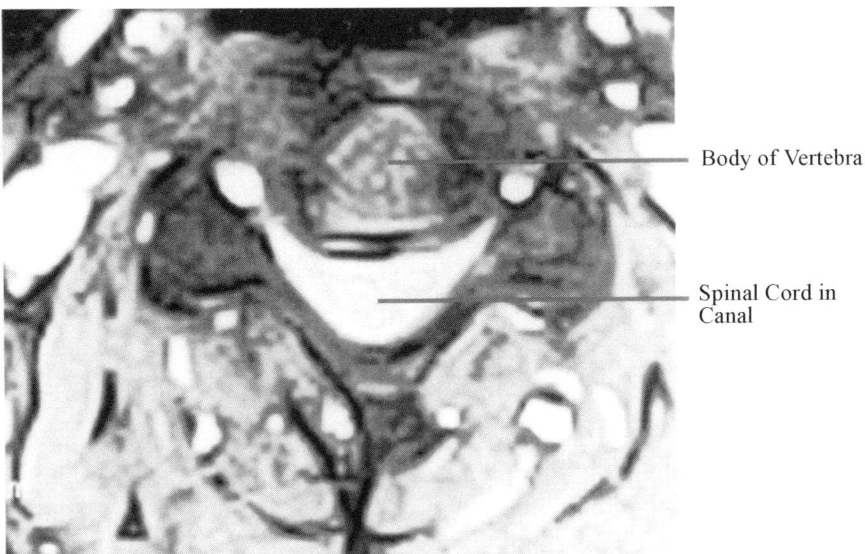

Figure 2.63   Computed tomography (axial plane).

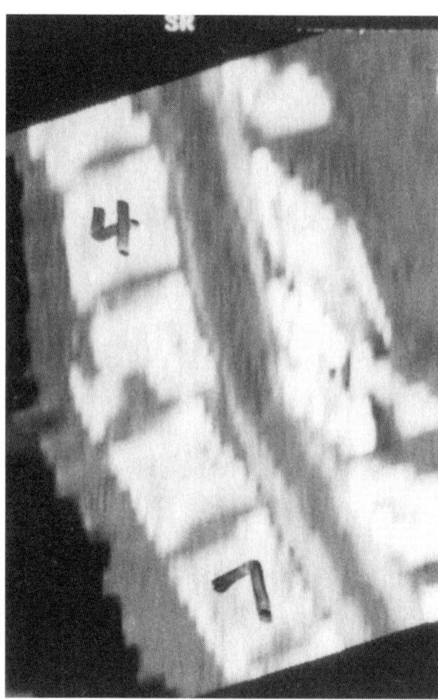

Figure 2.64   Reformatted CT (from axial to sagittal plane).

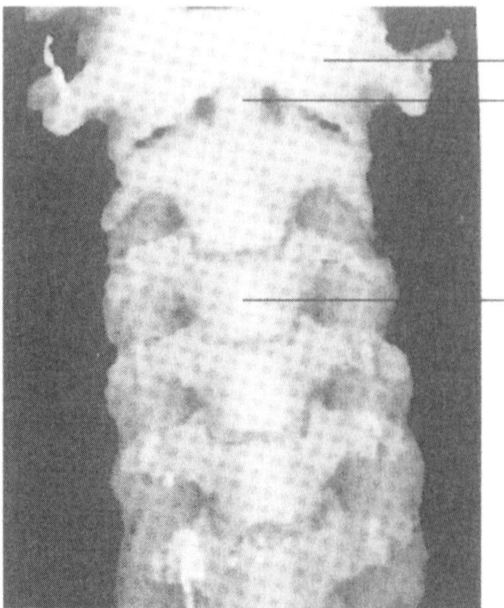

Figure 2.65   3-D CT of vertebral surface.   [Reproduced with permission.   Source: Harris, J.; Mirvis, S.   Radiology of Acute Cervical Spine Trauma, 3rd Edition. Williams & Wilkins (Baltimore), 1996.]

that, compared to conventional tomography, computed tomography has better resolution, requires less radiation, can usually be obtained more rapidly, and is more amenable to reformatting.

MAGNETIC RESONANCE IMAGING

Introduction

Magnetic resonance imaging (MRI or MR) (Figure 2.66), similar to CT, is a relatively new imaging modality that increasingly is being used to assess neck trauma. Unlike plain films or CT, however, MR does not require x-rays to obtain an image. Whereas both plain film and CT are based on x-ray transmission through the region being imaged, MR is based on emission, i.e., the imaging information is transmitted from the region of interest. Also, instead of x-rays, MR uses a combination of a magnetic field and a radio-frequency signal to obtain an image.

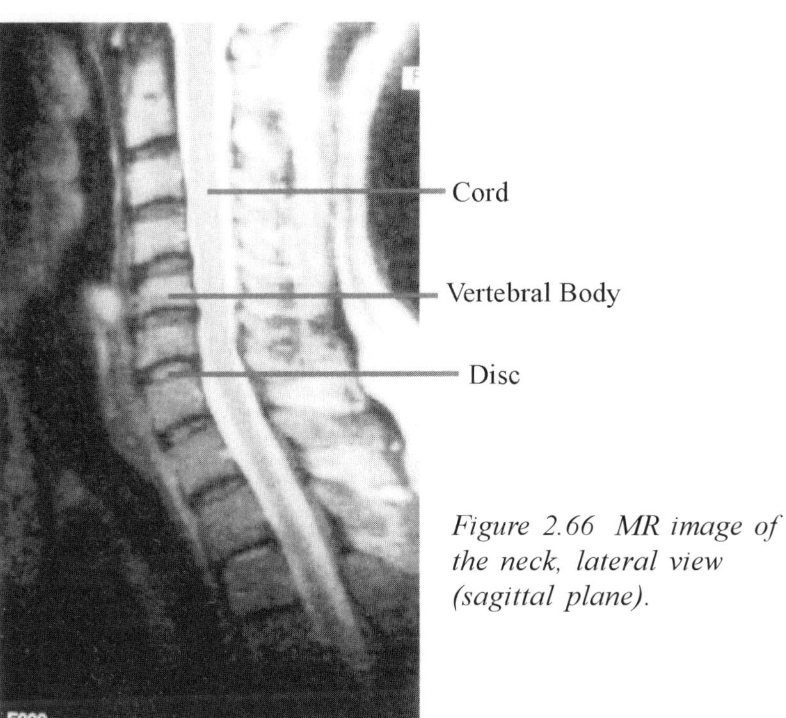

Figure 2.66 MR image of the neck, lateral view (sagittal plane).

MR is especially well suited to displaying soft tissue injuries, such as inter-vertebral disc herniation (Figure 2.67). Note that the disc distortion can be directly visualized on this sagittal view MR. (In contrast, recall that when using a sagittal view [lateral view] x-ray, the extrusion of disc material into the canal often has to be inferred, and the extent of extrusion is usually more difficult to assess.)

Discussion

To obtain an MR image of the neck, the subject is placed in a magnetic field, which is maintained while a radio frequency (RF) signal is rapidly switched on and off (an RF pulse). The two electromagnetic fields thus created interact with the atomic structure of the neck tissue to create the MR image. More specifically, the imaging depends on the magnetic properties of atomic nuclei.

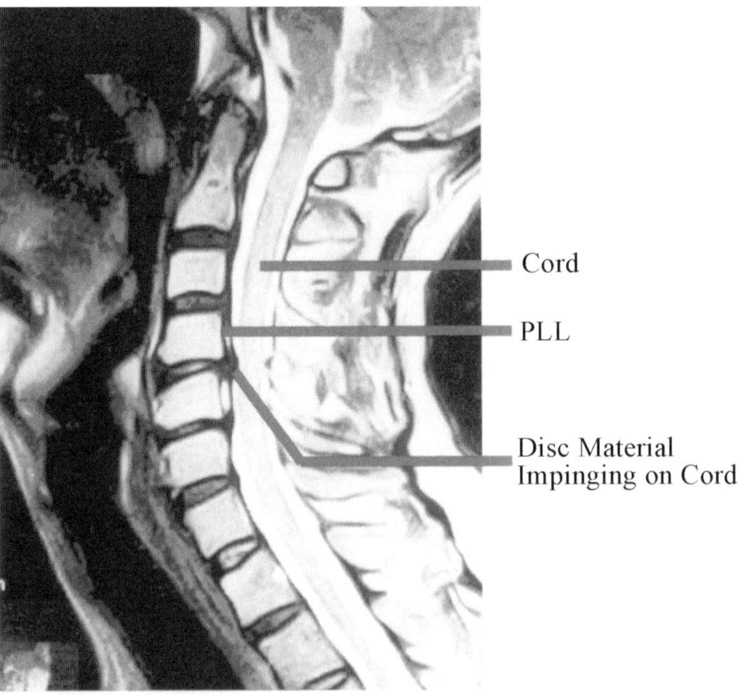

Figure 2.67 Disc herniation.

The nucleus of a hydrogen atom—a single proton—is characterized by a magnetic field and a "spin" (angular momentum). The magnetic field is a vector quantity and as such may be described in terms of its magnitude and direction. These two characteristics define the "magnetic moment" of the field.

The magnetic moment of the proton may be conceptualized as being associated with a very small magnet. This magnet is not stationary, however; it is rotating about its axis. Ordinarily, the magnetic fields due to protons in the human body are randomly arranged, and hence these fields cancel each other. Thus, when "viewed" from the "outside," there is no net magnetic field. However, in the presence of an external magnetic field, some of the magnetic moments will align themselves with the external magnetic field (much the way a compass needle aligns itself with the magnetic field of the earth) and thereby produce a net magnetic field.

In the presence of an external magnetic field, the magnetic moments will also precess (rotate, in a cone-like pattern, about the direction of the external field), and if exposed to a radio frequency pulse of the proper frequency,[16] the moments will nutate (i.e., tilt toward the axial plane). When the magnetic moments associated with individual nuclei precess at the same frequency as the radio pulse, they are said to be in resonance. Magnetic resonance is named for this resonance.

When the RF pulse is turned off, the protons stop tilting and return to their alignment with the magnetic field (which is still being applied). This return to the "forced" alignment of the protons with the external (axial) magnetic field is referred to as proton relaxation. (Although the protons are not really relaxed, in that they are still "forcefully" being lined up by the magnetic field, the terminology is perhaps somewhat similar to that used to describe a soldier being "at ease" after being at "attention.") This relaxation does not occur instantaneously, but rather at some rapid but finite rate, described by two time constants. The first time constant, T1 (spin-lattice relaxation), describes the increasing axial magnetization, whereas the second time constant, T2 (spin-spin relaxation), describes the decreasing transverse magnetization.

Typically, T1 is on the order of several tenths of a second, while T2 is on the order of several hundredths of a second (Hendee 1992). The growing axial magnetization and the decaying transverse magnetization correspond to

---

[16] The proper radio frequency, called the Larmor frequency, depends on a number of factors, including the strength of the magnetic field. For a magnetic field of 1.0 Tesla (a value typical for diagnostic imaging and equal to approximately 20,000 times the strength of the earth's magnetic field), the Larmor frequency is approximately 43 MHz.

different tissue properties. Two parameters, TR (the repetition time) and TE (the echo time), can be selected as part of the imaging process to produce an MR image that is "T1-weighted" or "T2-weighted" (Figures 2.68 and 2.69).

The two weightings may be used to form images that emphasize different injuries or may provide different indications of a given injury. For example, the T1-weighted image (Figure 2.68) depicts a rather small spinal cord hematoma (thereby pointing to cord injury), whereas a T2-weighted image (Figure 2.69) of the same patient, depicts rather extensive edema in the same region of the spinal cord (also pointing to cord injury).

The different weightings may also be used in two primary imaging sequences, referred to as GE (gradient-recalled echo) and SE (spin-echo imaging). Essentially, GE is used when quick imaging is required or to obtain dynamic images (e.g., blood flow), whereas SE imaging provides more anatomic detail but requires longer imaging time.

Although the magnetic field that is used to generate an MR image is not thought to be harmful per se, this field and the gantry-like structure used to generate it may place some indirect restrictions on the use of the technique. For example, the field may interfere with the proper operation of a pacemaker. Another example involves the interaction of the field with certain materials. The presence of so-called ferromagnetic material, such as that used to tie together adjacent vertebrae that are being surgically "fused" (e.g., after the disc separating them has been removed), may produce an artifact, thereby appearing to indicate an injury where there is none. T1-weighted imaging is sometimes used to reduce the effects of ferromagnetic materials on MR images (Hall 1993). Figure 2.70 shows both an actual injury and an artifact due to the presence of ferromagnetic material.

Another restriction on the use of MR is related to the structure used to generate the image. Traditionally, MR images have been obtained with the subject positioned in a rather confining cylindrical chamber. If a patient is claustrophobic, he or she may not be able to remain in the imaging chamber long enough for the image to be generated. However, new MR systems are being designed, which have less confining chambers.

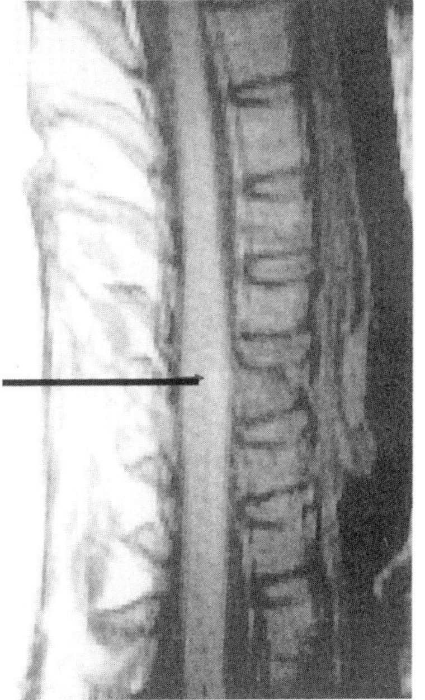

Figure 2.68 Spinal cord hematoma (T1-weighted MR). [Reproduced with permission. Source: Mirvis, S.E.; Young, J.W.R. Imaging in Trauma and Critical Care. *Williams & Wilkins (Baltimore), 1992.]*

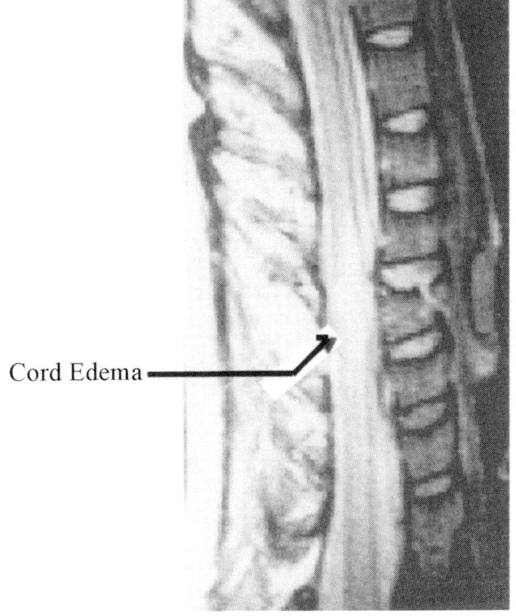

Figure 2.69 Spinal cord edema (T2-weighted MR). [Reproduced with permission. Source: Mirvis, S.E.; Young, J.W.R. Imaging in Trauma and Critical Care. *Williams & Wilkins (Baltimore), 1992.]*

Figure 2.70 MR artifact due to ferromagnetic material.

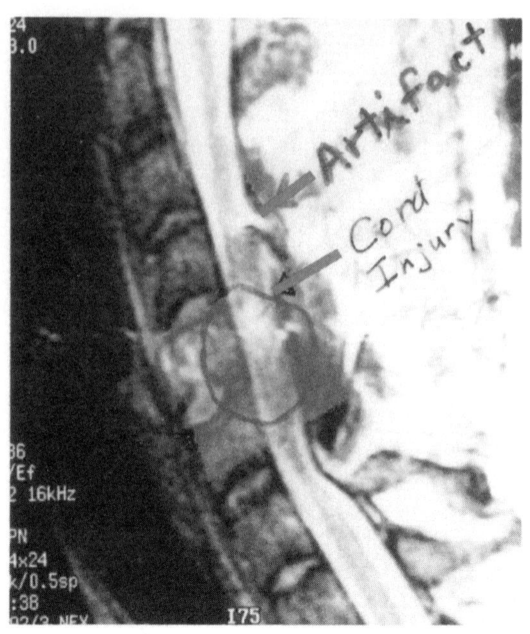

Chapter 3

Injuries and Injury Mechanisms

Jeffrey A. Pike
Frank A. Pintar
Narayan Yoganandan
Jeffrey S. Augenstein
Tristram Horton

Introduction

Categorization of Neck Injury

In addition to understanding injury mechanisms, it is important to understand the nature and consequences of different neck injuries. Traditionally, trauma to the cervical spine has been divided into three categories: (1) injury to osseous components (i.e., bones), (2) injury to neurological structures, and (3) injury to soft tissue support structures. The first category denotes fractures of the vertebral column. The second category includes trauma to the spinal cord and spinal nerves. The third category is concerned with ligamentous and muscular injury. This injury classification involves considerable overlap. For example, a fractured vertebra may involve spinal cord disruption as a result of bone fragment retropulsion into the spinal canal. Although not the focus of this text, the cervical spine may be affected by injuries to vascular and respiratory structures in the neck. These will also be touched on in the discussion.

Osseous Injury

Fractures are grouped according to the anatomical location of the injury within the vertebral column. Specifically, the injury may involve the anterior components (vertebral body and end plates) or the posterior components (pedicles, transverse processes, lateral masses, superior and inferior facets, laminae, and spinous processes). There are two primary concerns with cervical vertebral fractures: whether or not the fracture has resulted in impingement of neurological structures, and whether or not the fracture is structurally stable. It is important to note that most cervical spine fractures do not have neurological sequelae and are structurally stable. Determination of these factors is by clinical assessment and radiological analysis. A review of radiological assessment appears in Chapter 2.

Neurological Injury

Injury to the neurological elements of the cervical spine is generally the result of primary osseous injury (fracture) or soft tissue injury (for example, ligamentous disruption). This is the most severe class of neck injuries. Such injuries can result in spasticity, paresis, paralysis, long-term neck or referred pain, or even death.

Soft Tissue Injury

Soft tissue neck injury is the most common type of neck injury in the vehicular crash environment. Neck sprains, in which the ligaments have been stretched beyond their normal limits, are seen more often than any other spine injury. Generally, this injury is a result of flexion-extension (a so-called "whiplash" injury). Although such injuries are usually minor, when severe, ligamentous injury can include disruption of ligamentous structures with concomitant joint dislocation. This type of soft tissue injury is very dangerous and can impart severe neurological impairment.

In the vehicular crash environment, most neck injuries are due to neck movement rather than to direct contact with the neck. Therefore, an injury can be classified as being a flexion-type injury, an extension-type injury, and so on. The injurious motions can also occur in combination, giving rise to additional categories such as flexion plus rotation-type injury. The modifier "hyper" is sometimes added to the motion (e.g., hyperflexion injury) to denote motion that is in some sense excessive. In one sense, however, any injury-producing motion is excessive for the individual and circumstances involved. In addition to neck motion, forces, usually compressive or distractive, can be transmitted to the neck via the head and torso. For example, a flexed neck may receive compressive loading as a result of the top of the head impacting the roof of the vehicle.

Clinicians have generally advanced injury mechanisms based on retrospective analysis of patient x-rays and/or clinical evaluation. For example, if a vertebral body is crushed and severely reduced in height, one presumes that compressive force was responsible for the injury. Crash investigators have generally advanced injury mechanisms based on a retrospective analysis of the vehicle and roadway. For example, vehicle damage will give a good indication of where the vehicle was struck and hence how the occupant moved during the crash (in general, the occupant[s] will tend to move toward the impact location) and skid marks on the highway would indicate a certain amount of pre-crash awareness and slowing down before impact. With the development of multi-disciplinary accident investigation teams, retrospective studies involve a combination of roadway, vehicle, and occupant (including clinical) information.

The text includes examples of various injuries and injury mechanisms, as well as the associated vehicle crashes. These crashes may be described as low speed, medium speed, high speed, or very high speed, based primarily on the extent and nature of the vehicle damage. The crash is also characterized by the direction of the main force produced by the crash (the principal direction of force, or PDOF). This is expressed with reference to the face of a clock, e.g., a 2 o'clock PDOF. This can be thought of as describing the location that an occupant would move toward during the crash (until his or her trajectory is modified, e.g., by a restraint). Thus, in a "pure" frontal crash (12 o'clock PDOF), the occupant(s) move straight forward; in a pure rear-end crash (6 o'clock PDOF), the occupant(s) initially move straight backward.

One alternative way of establishing injury mechanisms is to conduct a laboratory investigation of particular kinds of injuries to the cervical spine. This has been done for some mechanisms, but not all cervical spine injury mechanisms have been completely evaluated. Although the injury mechanisms classified in the present chapter originate from clinical evaluation, experimental studies that have verified the stated injury mechanisms are referenced as well. The mechanism of injury of some specific types of trauma to the neck remains controversial, in part because of the lack of experimental validation of these specific injuries.

Injury to the neck also can be evaluated in terms of the effect of injury on the neck's "conduit" functions, namely, the transport of air to and from the lungs and blood to and from the head, and the transmission of electrical impulses between the brain and the rest of the body. Thus, neck injuries that affect the functioning of the trachea or of the cervical spinal cord may be extremely significant, even though the amount of physical damage per se may not be extensive. Conversely, there may be fairly extensive physical damage (e.g., fractured vertebra) without any significant effect on cord function.

Three characteristics of neck injury will be discussed in this chapter: (1) injury mechanism, (2) structure initially affected, and (3) severity of injury. These characteristics, in turn, can provide the basis for various biomechanical accident studies and lead to further improvements in driver, highway, and vehicle safety performance, as well as improved patient care.

INJURY MECHANISMS

Some clinicians have expanded upon the traditional injury mechanisms. In particular, flexion and extension are further specified according to whether there was compressive or distractive loading (Allen 1982; Chandler 1992). This system is labeled "mechanistic" and classifies neck injuries into six categories of tissue failure (viz., compressive flexion, distractive flexion, vertical compression, compressive extension, distractive extension, and lateral flexion). The categories are then subdivided into stages, with each successive stage corresponding to a level of increased severity. For example, within compressive flexion we have: Stage I—anterior-superior corner of vertebral body is rounded; Stage II—wedge fracture; Stage III—fracture fragment of anterior-inferior corner; Stage IV—slight posterior translation of posterior margin of vertebral body; Stage V—significant posterior displacement of vertebral body (Allen 1982; Allen 1989). The staging was oriented toward clinical application, namely, helping to determine whether a particular injury would be amenable to non-surgical treatment (Chandler 1992). Of the six categories, three were found to be the most common: compressive and distractive flexion and vertical compression. The remaining three are compressive and distractive extension and lateral flexion. A particularly noteworthy feature of vertical compression is that, of the six categories, it is the only one for which cord injury, if it occurs, is most likely due to cord impingement by a retropulsed vertebral fracture fragment (from a so-called "burst" fracture). For the remaining five categories, if cord injury does occur, it is most likely due to ligament failure and the resulting vertebral displacement (Allen 1989).

Some clinicians still feel that there are advantages to the traditional, "older" system (Harris 1993), and it is not clear if one or the other will emerge as "the" system. This text will draw upon the mechanistic system but will primarily use the simpler, better-established nomenclature. The text will follow an anatomical organization, beginning superiorly and proceeding inferiorly along the cervical spinal column.

Although forces may cause the neck to undergo a particular motion overall (e.g., extension), portions of the neck may undergo different motions. For example, the C3/C4 segment (vertebrae C3 and C4, and the disc between them) may undergo extension, and the C5/C7 segment may undergo flexion. A portion of the vertebral column that undergoes a particular motion can be referred to as a motion segment.

Another effect that may occur is that two segments/regions may both be undergoing flexion, but one may have compressive loading, while the other has distractive loading. It is relatively common for compressive flexion and distractive flexion to occur during the same event. When this occurs, it is likely that the compression and distraction motion segments will be contiguous, with the distractive segment being superior and the compressive segment being inferior (Allen 1989).

When studying spinal injury mechanisms and/or repair, it is often useful to consider the vertebral column not as a single column but rather as being composed of two or three sub-columns. The two-column concept originated about 50 years ago (Nicoll 1949; Roaf 1960; Holdsworth 1963) and remains in use today.

The two-column concept (Figure 3.1) essentially divides the vertebral column into anterior and posterior segments. The anterior column consists of the anterior longitudinal ligament (ALL), vertebral body, disc, and posterior longitudinal ligament (PLL). The posterior column consists of the posterior elements, i.e., all other spinal structures.

The three-column concept (Figure 3.2) essentially subdivides the anterior column of the two-column model into an anterior and a middle column. The three-column concept was originally applied to the thoracolumbar spine (Denis 1983) and has been adapted for the cervical spine and incorporated into the mechanistic classification of spinal injury. In the three-column concept, the columns are defined as follows (Allen 1989; Stauffer 1991):

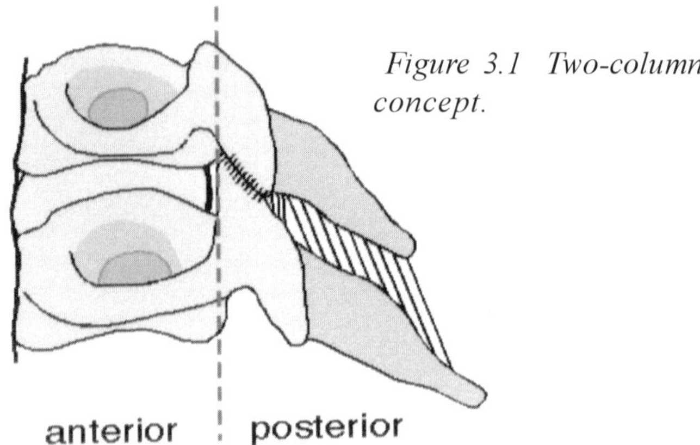

Figure 3.1   Two-column concept.

Anterior: Anterior longitudinal ligament, anterior half of disc,
             anterior half of vertebral body.
Middle: Posterior longitudinal ligament, posterior half of disc,
             posterior half of vertebral body.
Posterior: Vertebral arches and supporting ligaments.

The ligaments associated with each of the three columns can then be referred to as the anterior, mid-, and posterior ligament complexes, and mechanical stability can then be defined in terms of failure of the middle ligament complex (Clintron 1981; Jofe 1989; White 1990). As a practical

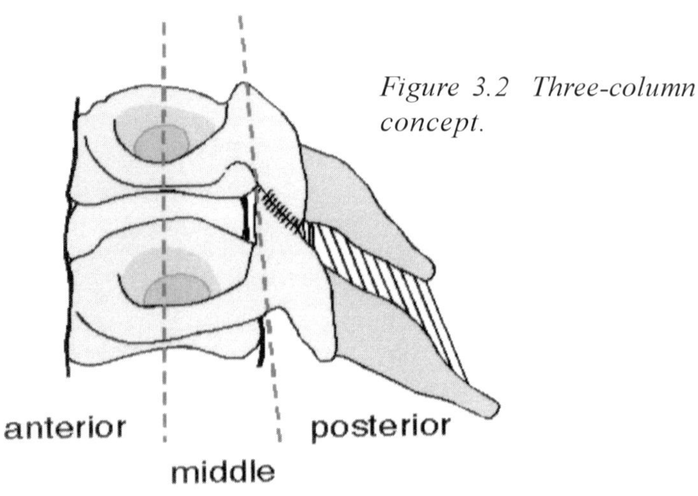

Figure 3.2   Three-column concept.

matter, this means an injury involving the middle ligament complex plus at least one of the other two ligament complexes. Stability has also been defined in other terms, including: interspinous angulation >11 degrees; A-P translation >3.5 mm; or disc space separation >1.7 mm (White 1990).

STRUCTURE INJURED

Spinal structures that may be injured include the vertebra, ligaments, discs, and the surrounding soft tissue. Injury mechanisms in the vehicular crash environment (i.e., blunt, non-penetrating trauma) may include direct neck impact. However, most of the injuries that will be discussed here are due to various neck motions (e.g., flexion, extension, and combinations such as flexion plus rotation). Perhaps the most important categorization of a given neck injury is whether or not the spinal cord has been injured (or is likely to be injured).

Injury to the anterior region of the neck may be due to either direct contact (e.g., with a steering wheel rim) or neck motion (e.g., extension). Injuries to the spinal cord, in the vehicular crash environment, are precipitated by other injuries, usually to nearby structures. In the cervical region, the most prevalent cord injury mechanism is via the relative translation of adjacent vertebrae, whereby the cord is trapped and compressed, and/or stretched (Figure 3.3).

Soft Tissue Neck Trauma

There are many important structures in the front of the neck (see Chapter 1), including the thyroid and cricoid cartilage and the larynx. Although these may be injured via neck motion, they are more vulnerable to direct contact such as with the steering wheel rim. In particular, the thyroid cartilage (the Adam's apple) is in a prominent location and has a low fracture force (typically <445 N [100 lb]) (SAE 1986).

Cartilage fractures are typical of other injuries to structures of the neck, in that the injuries may not be especially significant in and of themselves, but because of their proximity to the airway and to the cerebral vasculature, they may interfere with airway patency (i.e., breathing) and/or carotid blood flow (blood supply to the brain). As mentioned previously, direct impact is not the only way that anterior structures of the neck may be injured. As the following discussion indicates, they may also be injured by neck motion.

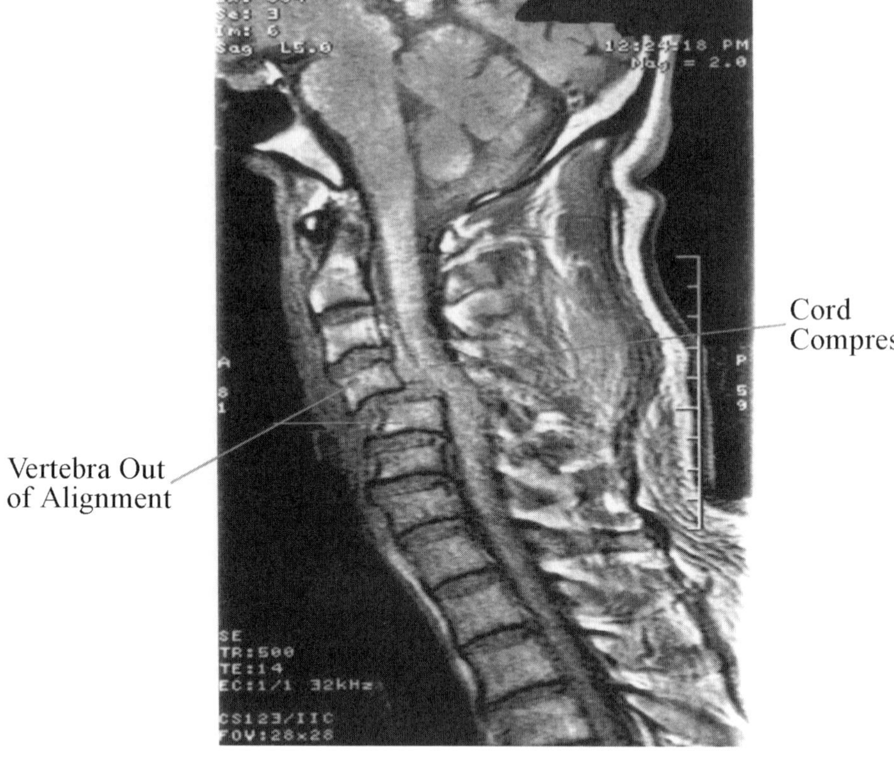

Figure 3.3   Cord injury from vertebral movement.

Cervical Sprain

Under non-injurious conditions, the muscles, tendons, and ligaments of the neck will stretch to accommodate neck movement. When the neck returns to its neutral position, these soft tissue structures will conform to their pre-stretch shape. This includes the joint capsules, the ligamentous envelopes that enclose each disc and each facet joint. If neck movement is such that the soft tissue is stretched beyond its elastic limit, it will not return to its original shape and size, even when the stretching is discontinued. This is sometimes referred to as plastic (as opposed to elastic) deformation. If the stretching continues beyond this point, the tissue begins to tear. The soft tissues involved most often are the muscles attached to the vertebrae and/or the ligamentous structures that connect two or more vertebrae. When the ligaments and/or neck muscles stretch to the point of minor tearing, it is often referred to as cervical sprain.

Although ligament tears per se can be painful, a ligament injury becomes of even greater concern if it affects the ability of the ligament to maintain the relative position of adjacent vertebrae. Ligamentous injury may not produce neurological sequelae at the instant of trauma but may permit subsequent neurological injury. The ability of the ligaments to prevent (additional) injury after initial trauma is addressed in the concept of stability. Basically, an injury may be considered stable if subsequent daily activities are not likely to produce any (additional) neurological consequences.

Trauma may also deform one or more of the intervertebral discs. If the deformation is sufficient, the disc may tear or even rupture. Similar to the concerns regarding vertebral fracture, a major concern regarding a torn or ruptured disc is whether the disc will bulge rearward, or whether the nucleus pulposus (the gelatinous filling of the disc) will be extruded rearward (retropulsed) and press on a spinal nerve or spinal nerve root (branches of the spinal cord), or possibly even press on the spinal cord itself (Figure 3.4). Depending on the extent and nature of the intrusion into the neural tissue, some pain or loss of sensation or even paralysis may result.

A ligament may also push against the cord. This is particularly true in the elderly, in whom the ligamenta flavum is prone to buckle (Hockberger 1988) and, during neck extension, may push against the cord and produce an injury to the inner diameter of the cord (Duckworth 1984). This injury, called central cord syndrome, is discussed later in this chapter.

It is worth emphasizing that a vertebral fracture per se is not sufficient to cause neurological deficit. Indeed, approximately 60% of cervical fractures have no associated neurological injury (Mahoney 1988). Thus, a so-called broken neck (fracture of one or more cervical vertebrae), although serious in its own right, becomes much more severe if the bone is broken in such a way that the bone then injures the spinal cord (Figure 3.5).

Factors Affecting Injury

The various injuries already discussed here frequently are due NOT to some unique loading and movement that is absent in non-injurious motion, but rather are due to extremes of the various loadings and movements that are part of

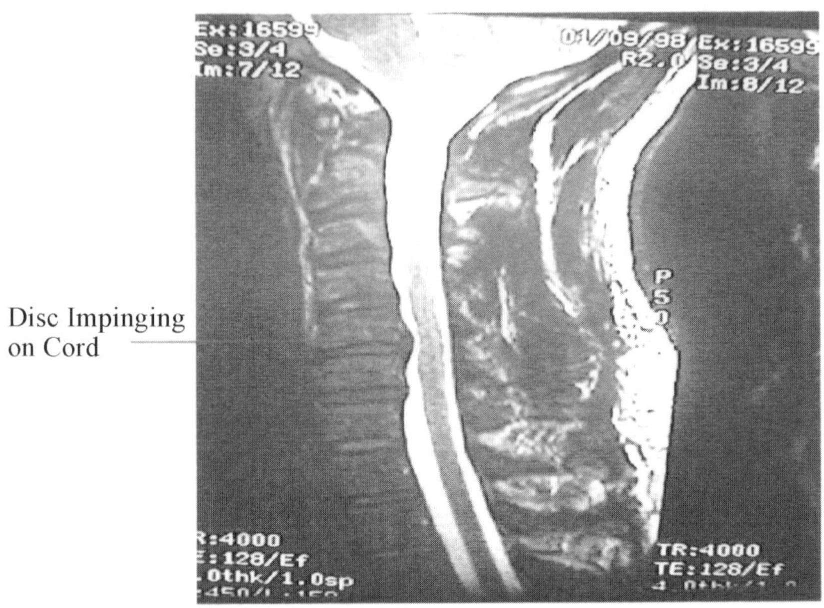

Disc Impinging on Cord

Figure 3.4   Herniated disc impinging on cord at C5-C6 (MRI).

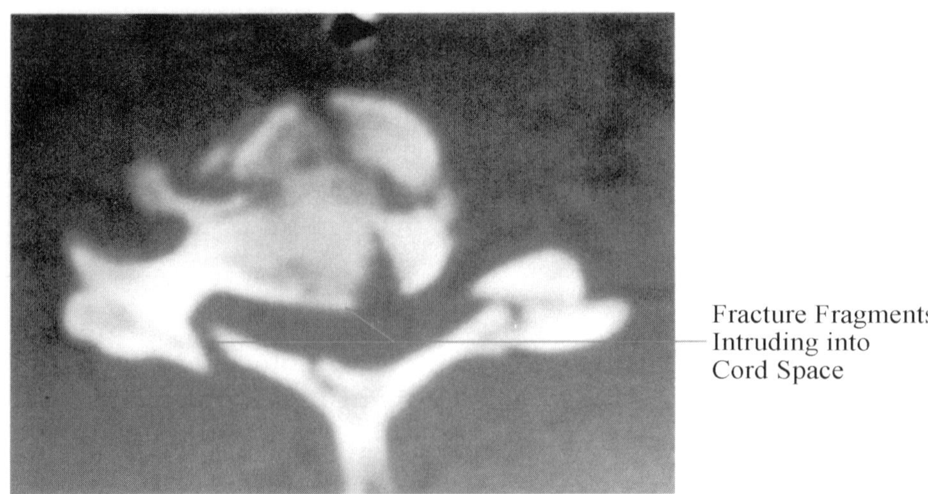

Fracture Fragments Intruding into Cord Space

Figure 3.5   Vertebral fracture with cord injury.

the normal functioning of the spine. These include distraction (tension), compression, flexion, extension, lateral flexion (lateral bending), rotation, and combinations thereof. Clearly, there are a great many different combinations of the various motions; therefore, the spine can be injured as the result of a great many different complex motions. Furthermore, more than one of these can occur during a single event (e.g., vehicle crash, fall) (Chandler 1992). Another important factor in neck injury is the "initial condition," i.e., the neck position at the time of loading (Hochberger 1988; Myers 1991; Pintar 1995; Yoganandan 1989). For example, whether the neck is in flexion, extension, or straight at the time of compressive loading will be a factor in determining the type of injury produced. As another example, consider that head impact may produce flexion-type injuries when the head/neck/thorax is pre-positioned to produce motion that is not mid-sagittal (e.g., the head is turned to the right or left and then flexion occurs), and these injuries may not occur if motion is limited to the mid-sagittal plane (Nusholtz 1981; Nusholtz 1983). Additionally, researchers report that a small change (1 cm; 0.4 in.) in the location of a head impact can produce a major change in the resultant injury (McElhaney 1983). As the following quotation from the White and Panjabi (White 1990) biomechanics text indicates, many factors help to determine which injuries, if any, are produced in a given crash:

> The load magnitude, the rate and duration of load application (the time history), the point of load application, the direction of loading, and the initial cervical spine position and relative positions of the head and thorax all determine the individual cervical spine injury.

Note that injury to the cord might be temporary, with some or perhaps all of the symptoms resolving over time. This concept of temporary versus permanent cord injury is discussed in Chapter 1. A number of injuries, arranged according to anatomical location, will now be discussed.

Upper Cervical Region (C0–C2)

Atlanto-Occipital Dislocation

The arrangement of the occipital condyles and the superior articular facets of the atlas permit significant flexion and extension in the sagittal plane (head nodding). However, very little lateral bending and no rotation will occur at this joint when it is intact. Dislocation occurs as a result of hyperextension, which tears some anterior structures—typically the tectorial and anterior atlanto-occipital membranes (Figure 3.6). The dislocation usually results in anterior displacement of the occipital condyles in relation to the superior articular facets of the atlas. In most cases, this injury is immediately fatal.

Case Study. A lap and shoulder restrained 37-year-old male driving a 1992 mid-size car was traveling in the wrong direction on a three-lane roadway. His vehicle collided head-on with a 1998 minivan, which was carrying eight occupants. The impact was front-to-front and at very high speed, with 75% right front to right front overlap (Figure 3.7). The subject vehicle, the car, was not equipped with air bags. The driver of the subject vehicle expired at the scene and was found sitting in the driver's seat, with restraints on, by police and EMS personnel. At autopsy, the subject was found to have an atlanto-occipital dislocation with associated cord contusion. He sustained multiple other injuries including maxillary and nasal bone fractures as well as multiple facial contusions and lacerations. The mechanism of injury to the cranio-cervical junction, dictated by the occupant kinematics, involves hyperextension. Upon impact, the subject initially tended to move straight ahead. His restraints limited his forward motion and prevented contact of his torso with the steering column or instrument panel of his vehicle. After his torso was stopped, his head continued forward motion, until facial contact with the steering wheel produced a translational force causing extension at the occipito-atlantal joint with concomitant sheering. This series of events resulted in complete disruption of the occipito-atlantal ligament complex and C0/C1 dislocation.

Compression Fracture of C1

As discussed previously, the structure of C1 is unique, so it is not surprising that its fracture pattern is also somewhat unique. The term "burst fracture," when applied to C1, refers to a fracture of both the anterior and posterior arches (Figure 3.8). Burst fractures of C1 were studied in great detail by Dr. Jefferson in the early 1900s; thus, burst fractures of C1 are frequently referred to as "Jefferson" fractures. As originally described by Dr. Jefferson, the C1 fractures were bilateral in both the anterior and posterior arches of C1 (Jefferson 1920).

A - Apical Ligament
AAOM - Anterior Atlanto-Occipital Membrane
ALL - Anterior Longitudinal Ligament
B - Basion
C1 - Ring of Atlas
C2-VB – Vertebral Process of Axis
C2-SP – Spinous Process of Axis
D - Dens Process of Axis
M - Medulla
O - Opisthion
PAOM - Posterior Atlanto-Occipital Membrane
PLL - Posterior Longitudinal Ligament
T - Transverse Ligament

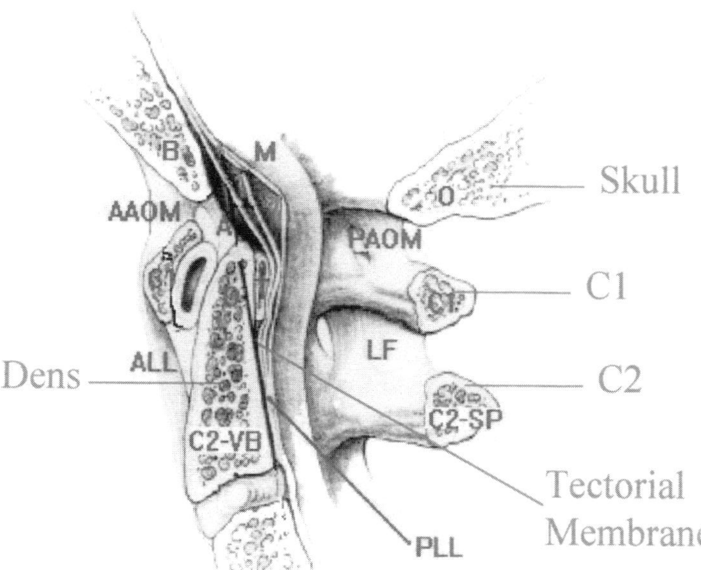

Figure 3.6   C0-C2 lateral view.

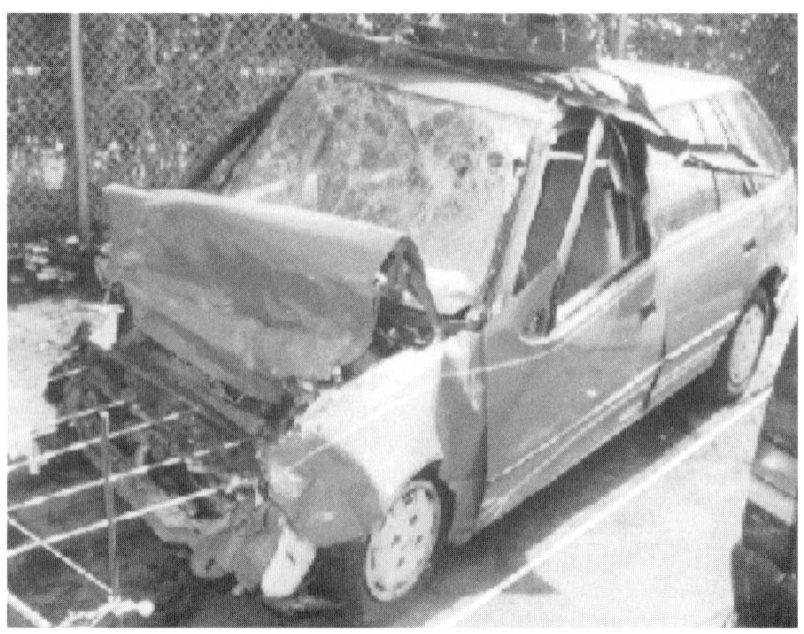

Figure 3.7 Case Study I—Subject vehicle.

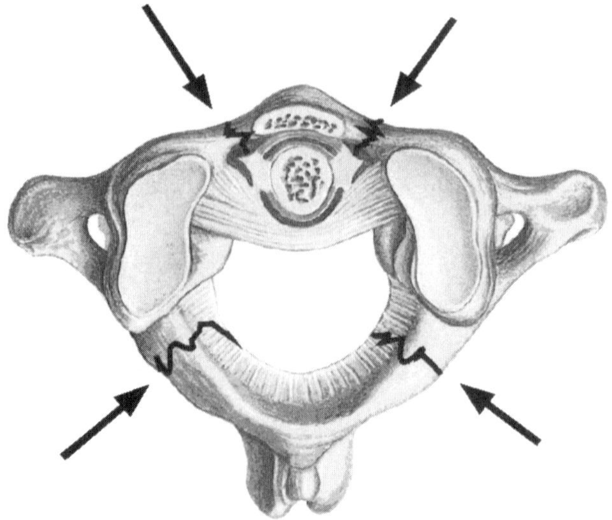

Figure 3.8 Burst fracture of C1 (Jefferson fracture).

Subsequent study with improved diagnostic equipment such as CT has shown that burst fractures of C1 always include at least one fracture of both the anterior and posterior arch, but need not be bilateral for either arch (Harris 1996). The geometry of the articular surfaces involved in the C0/C1 joint causes the fracture fragments to be outwardly displaced, i.e., moving away from the spinal canal. This, in concert with the fact that the structural integrity of the joint is normally not affected, results in little risk of neurological involvement. Injuries of this type are generally stable and heal well with minimal intervention.

The transverse atlantal ligament (Figure 3.9) may be disrupted in conjunction with a Jefferson fracture. If disrupted, the injury generally is unstable; if not disrupted, the injury generally is stable. An important exception to this rule occurs if a vertical (superior-inferior, or S-I oriented) fracture of one or both of the articular masses of C1 is associated with the bursting fracture of C1. Perhaps somewhat counterintuitively, the fracture may be more serious (unstable) if the articular mass fragments remain together. If the fracture splits the pillar into lateral and medial fragments, but the fragments are not pulled apart, it is an indication that the transverse atlantal ligament has been disrupted. If this is the case, the injury is unstable (White and Panjabi 1990). (If the ligament remained intact, it would transmit the avulsing force to its attachment point with C1 and thereby pull the fragments apart.)

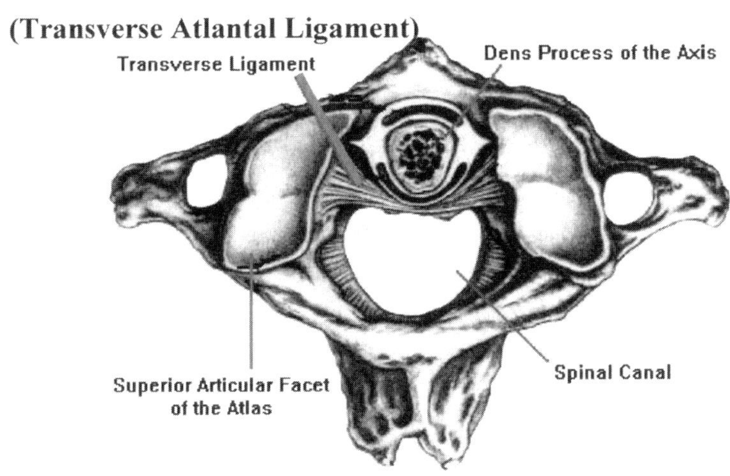

Figure 3.9 C1/C2 showing transverse atlantal ligament.

An open mouth view is frequently used to help visualize a burst fracture of C1. In this view, the fracture is typically characterized by an essentially symmetrical, lateral displacement of the articular masses (Figure 3.10). A similar depiction may be obtained with an A-P tomogram. An exception to this generalization is likely if the axial loading is not in the mid-sagittal plane, but rather is off-center. In such a case, both pillars would still be displaced laterally, but the pillar that is contralateral to the impact site may demonstrate more displacement.

Atlas Fracture—Anterior

Fractures may, of course, affect any part of C1. Fracture of the front part of the ring, i.e., the anterior arch of C1, is relatively rare. One way anterior arch fracture may occur is as an avulsion fracture; the anterior atlantoaxial ligament (AAOL), a caudal continuation of the anterior longitudinal ligament (ALL)

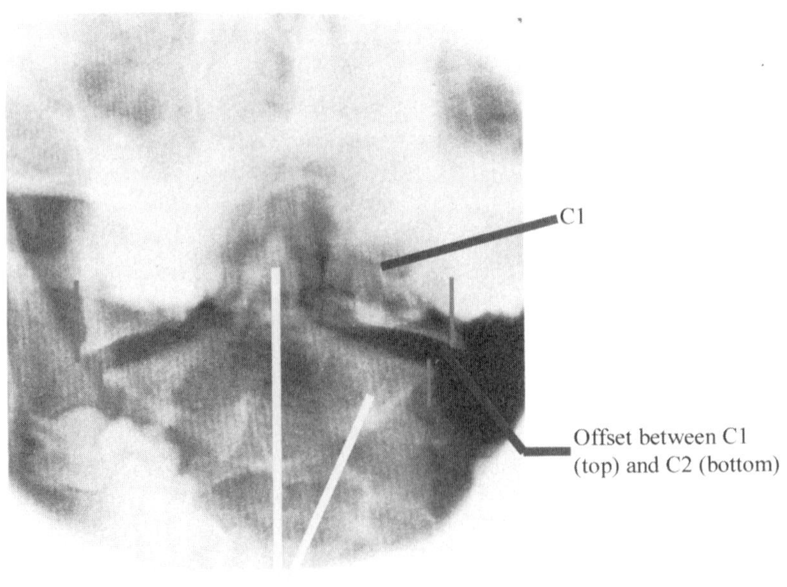

Figure 3.10 Burst fracture of C1. [Reproduced with permission. Source: Greenspan, A. Orthopedic Radiology—A Practical Approach, 2nd Edition. Lippincott-Raven (Philadelphia), 1997.]

(Figure 3.6), remains intact and exerts enough tensile force on C1 to fracture it (Clemente 1985). In this instance, the fracture is transverse, the ligament remains intact, and the posterior arch of C1 remains intact. The injury does not produce any neurological deficit, and the spine remains structurally stable. (The AAOL is a cranial continuation of the anterior longitudinal ligament that helps connect C1 and C2. More specifically, the AAOL connects the inferior border of the anterior arch of C1 to the anterior surface of the body of C2.)

Atlas Fracture—Posterior

Although the posterior atlas fracture may seem like a very logical "reciprocal" of the anterior atlas fracture just discussed, these fractures are actually quite different. First, this is a relatively common injury, whereas the anterior atlas fracture is relatively rare. Second, the mechanism of injury is quite different. The posterior atlas fracture is generally not an avulsion injury, but rather is produced by the compressive forces developed by neck extension when the atlas is compressed between C0 (the skull) and C2. Also unlike the anterior arch fracture, the posterior arch fracture typically involves fracture of both the left and right sides of the arch and disruption of the transverse atlantal ligament (Harris 1996). Similar to the anterior atlas fracture, the posterior atlas fracture is also generally mechanically stable and does not produce neurological deficit.

Atlanto-Axial Fracture—Dislocation

Injury at the C1-2 joint may involve dislocation with or without fracture of the bony elements. A variety of different mechanisms have been identified for these injuries, including hyperflexion, hyperextension, and either of these motions coupled with rotation.

Odontoid Fractures

Fracture of the odontoid process (dens) of the axis (C2) is relatively common, accounting for approximately 10% of all cervical fractures (Levy 1986). Although the odontoid may be fractured by flexion, extension, or occasionally even lateral flexion, flexion fractures of the odontoid are the most common (Anderson 1989). A commonly used system for categorizing fractures of the odontoid process is based on the location of the fracture (Anderson 1974). In this system, three types of dens fractures are denoted.

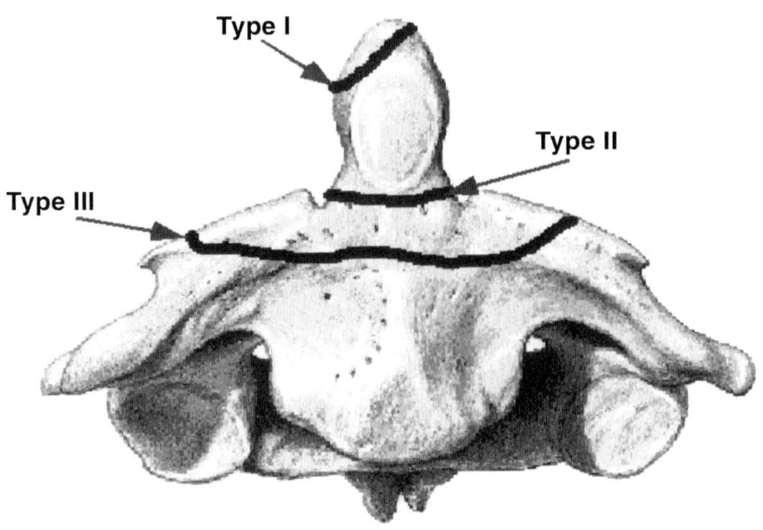

Figure 3.11   Three types of dens fractures.

A Type I dens fracture refers to an oblique fracture of the superior region of the dens (Figure 3.11). This fracture is relatively rare, accounting for only approximately 5% of dens fractures (Orrison 1989). When a Type I dens fracture does occur, it is typically an avulsion fracture, i.e., the tip of the dens is pulled off by force transmitted via the alar ligament (Figure 3.12), which is attached to the dens at this location.

The Type II fracture is the most common of the three, accounting for approximately 65% of dens fractures (Orrison 1989). A Type II dens fracture occurs at the base of the dens (Figure 3.11), and the fracture line may be oblique or horizontal. If relatively horizontal, the fracture line may not be evident on axial CT. Although the "open mouth" plain film is especially well suited to visualizing this region, this particular fracture may be quite subtle on this view. In this instance, thin-slice CT and reconstructed CT views (Figure 3.13) may be used. A Type II dens fracture is usually accompanied by pre-vertebral soft tissue swelling. If the "fragment," i.e., the dens, is displaced anteriorly, the injury is thought to result from flexion. If the dens is displaced posteriorly, the injury is thought to result from extension (Anderson 1989). Type II dens fractures are considered unstable. It is fairly common for the Type II dens fracture not to heal properly; that is, the fragment does not structurally reunite with the rest of the axis. The non-union rate for all Type II fractures is on the order of

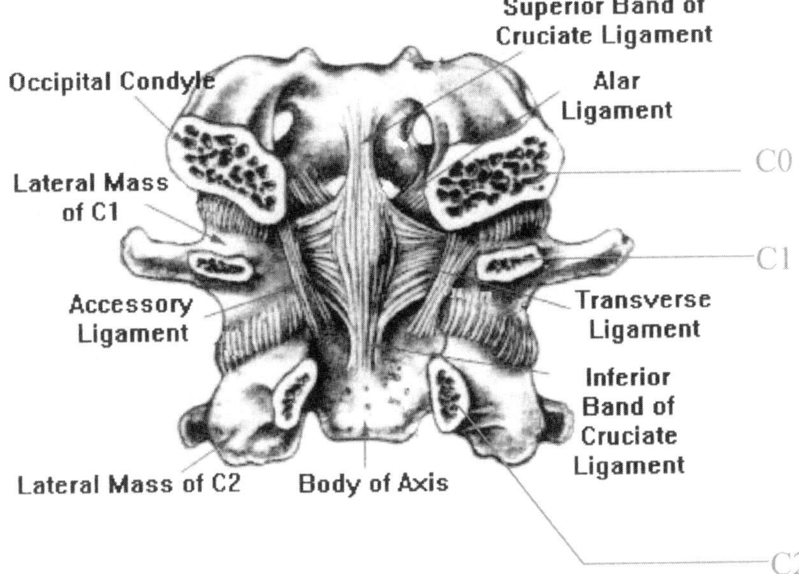

Figure 3.12   C0-C2, posterior cutaway view.

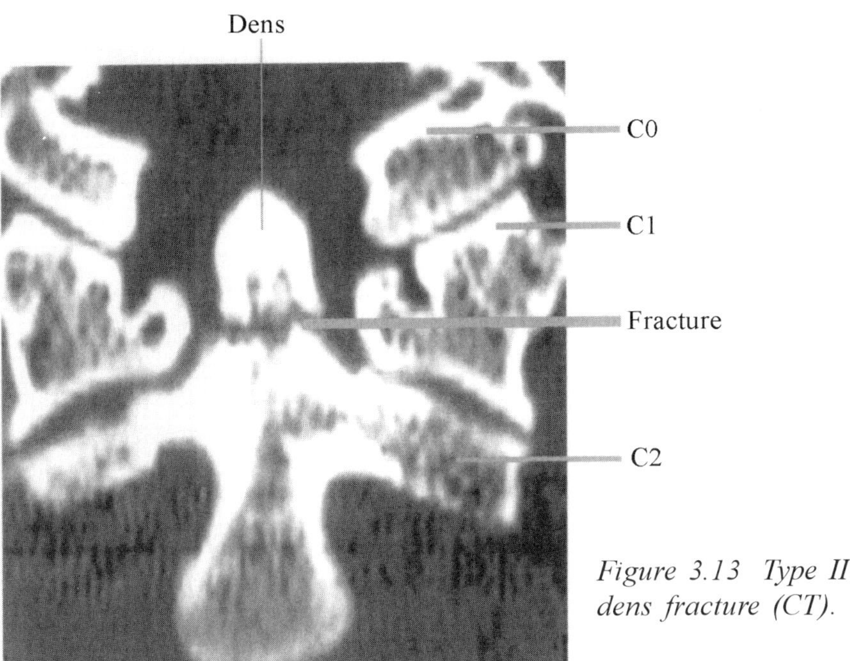

Figure 3.13   Type II dens fracture (CT).

50% (Barr 1988), with the highest rate of non-union for those fractures with the dens displaced posteriorly (Anderson 1989). This condition of a non-reunited dens fracture is referred to as os odontoidium. It should be noted that os odontoidium has been observed in children who have had no history of cervical trauma (Harris 1996). Thus, in some instances, os odontoidium may be congenital rather than traumatic, or may be due to previously asymptomatic trauma. Regardless of the origin, the injury has the potential for (additional) spinal cord trauma and thus is considered unstable.

The Type III dens fracture goes through the body of the axis (Figure 3.11) and hence is not actually a dens fracture, but rather a fracture of the body of the axis, near the dens-body junction. Type III fractures are about half as common as Type II fractures; thus, the Type III accounts for approximately one-third of all dens fractures (Orrison 1989). (Note: Due to the rarity of Type I fractures, dens fractures are sometimes simply classified as high or low—high referring to Type II, and low referring to Type III.)

The Type III fracture involves mostly soft, spongy cancellous bone, which heals much more readily than the hard, dense cortical bone of the dens itself. Therefore, non-union, for a Type III dens fracture, is unlikely. The Type III fracture usually involves at least one of the superior articulating facets as well. The fracture may be displaced; if it is, the injury may be unstable. If not displaced, the injury is considered to be stable. If there is neurological involvement, it most likely will involve mild upper extremity weakness, or Brown-Sequard syndrome (Galli 1989).

Occasionally, an odontoid fracture may occur during lateral flexion. When it does, most typically it is a Type III odontoid fracture and is produced via excessive loading of the atlas on the axis on the concave side of the laterally flexed spine. An oblique loading force applied to the head on one side causes lateral flexion of the neck. Consequently, a large compressive force is applied by the lateral mass of the atlas to the superior facet of the axis. The excessive lateral flexion with associated rotation results in fracture of the body, lateral mass, and transverse process of the axis on the concave side of the flexion. The lateral mass and transverse process fractures are a result of excessive force applied to this structure by the anterior lip of the superior facet of C3. Rotation is normally limited by contact between these elements. An example of this injury mechanism is provided in the following case study:

> **Case Study.** A 45-year-old unrestrained male was driving a 1996 mid-size passenger car when he was struck on the right side by a 1989 mid-size passenger car (Figure 3.14). The direction of the force

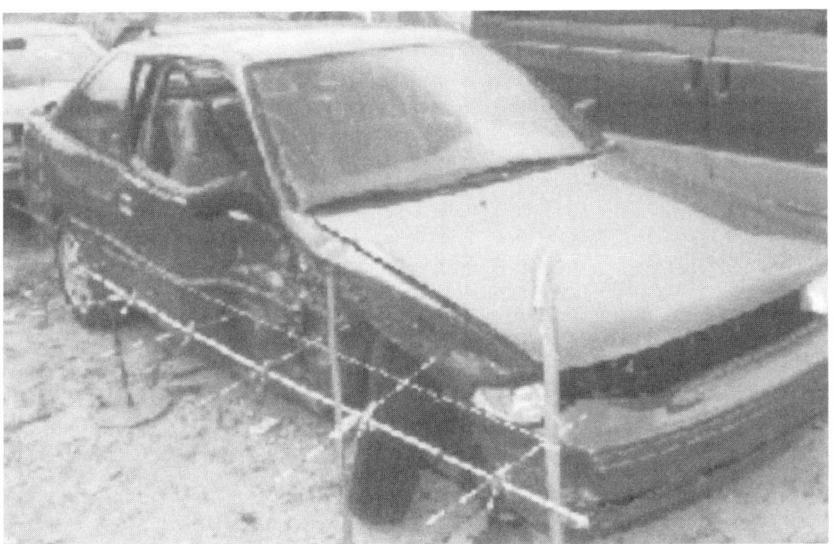

Figure 3.14   Case Study II—Subject vehicle.

of the impact (referred to as the principal direction of force, or PDOF) was 1 o'clock. (With reference to the face of a clock oriented so that 12 is straight ahead for the subject vehicle, the force of this crash acted as if it were applied from the 1 o'clock direction. Hence, the force tended to move the occupant toward the 1 o'clock location.) (Figure 3.15) The collision was of moderate severity. The subject was the lone occupant in the 1996 vehicle. Upon EMS arrival to the scene, the subject was found to be unresponsive and in respiratory arrest. He was intubated and transported to the hospital. At the hospital, he was found to have sustained a Type III odontoid fracture with posterior retropulsion of the C2-3 disc (Figure 3.16). This neck injury resulted in C2-level quadriplegia. The subject also sustained a minor upper forehead abrasion. He expired four months later. Autopsy examination indicated the extreme compression of the spinal cord (Figure 3.17). Type III odontoid fractures, as previously shown, are particularly worrisome, as the mechanism producing the fracture may result in ligamentous disruption and disc and/or bone fragment retropulsion with serious neurological sequelae.

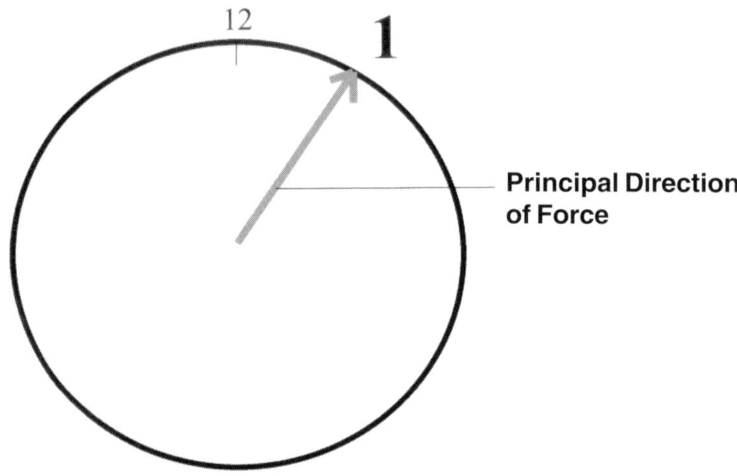

Figure 3.15   Case Study II—One o'clock principal direction of force (PDOF).

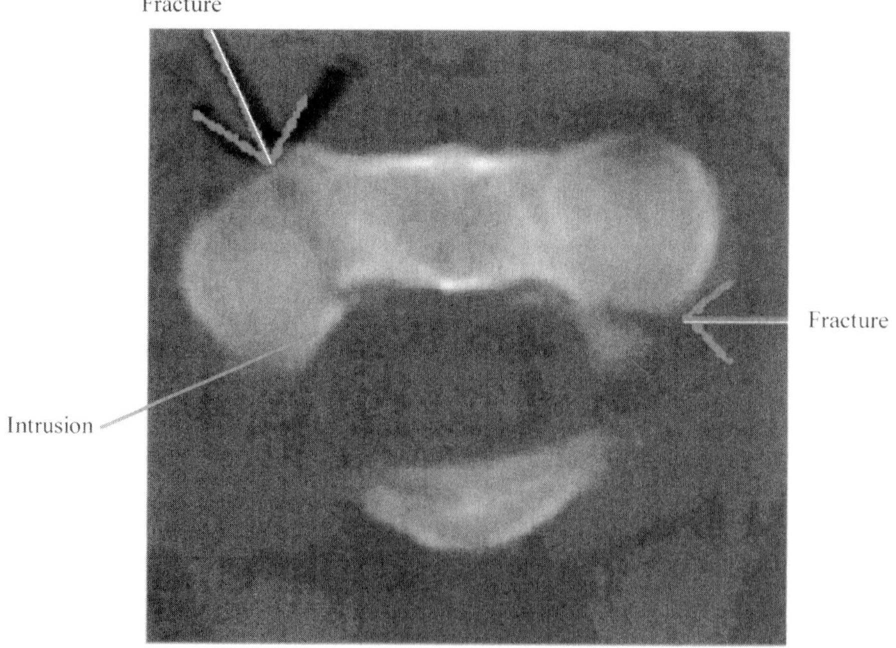

Figure 3.16   Case Study II—Type III dens fracture with canal intrusion.

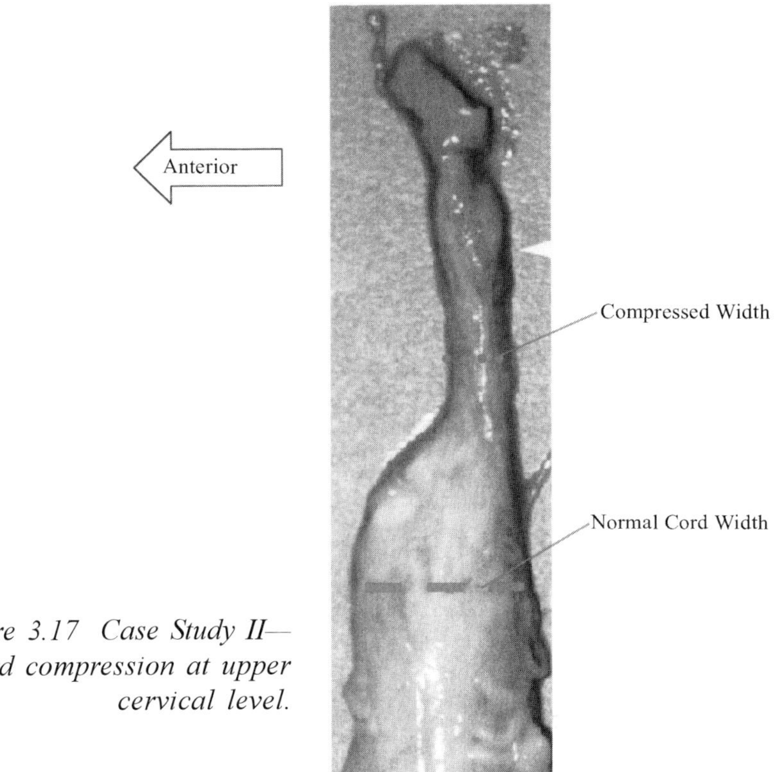

Figure 3.17 Case Study II— Cord compression at upper cervical level.

It has also been proposed that the magnitude of displacement is an important characteristic of the dens fracture, in that a dens fracture with a displacement of >5 mm (0.02 in.) tends to be less likely to achieve union than fractures with <5 mm displacement (Benson 1988; White 1990). Note that a dens fracture is often accompanied by a fracture of C1 (Benson 1988).

Axis Fracture

Extension may produce injury to the various regions of the axis (C2), including the lamina, the pars interarticularis, and the body. Laminar fracture generally occurs when a lamina is compressed between the laminae of contiguous vertebrae, i.e., the suprajacent and subjacent vertebrae. (This fracture was already discussed for C1, in which case it is referred to as "an [isolated] fracture of the posterior arch of C1.") Fractures of the pars or the body will now be discussed.

Hangman's Fracture

The region of the C2 pillars between the superior and inferior articular facets is named the pars interarticularis or, more simply, the isthmus. Thus, a C2 pillar fracture may be referred to as a pars interarticularis fracture or an isthmus fracture. This fracture may also be referred to by an assortment of other names, including traumatic spondylolisthesis of the axis. If the fracture is bilateral, the fracture is often referred to as a hangman's fracture (Figure 3.18).

Although the hangman's fracture nomenclature is quite picturesque, it is somewhat misleading. Judicial hanging typically produces bilateral pedicle fracture, but judicial hanging also produces distraction and shearing forces, which do not usually accompany the extension produced in vehicular crashes. The judicial "hangman's fracture" is a fracture-dislocation of the C1-2 joint in which a

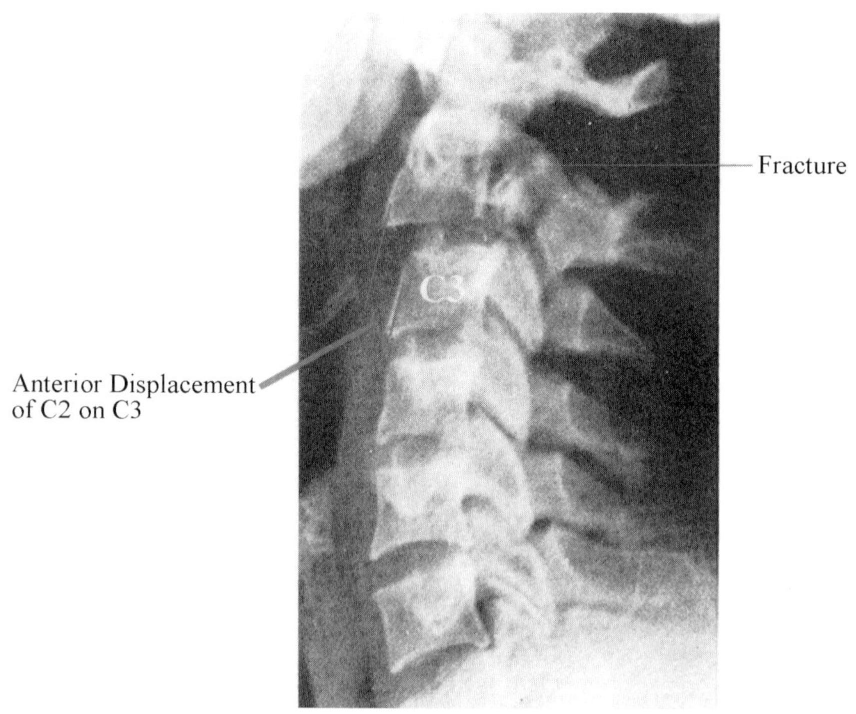

Figure 3.18 Hangman's fracture.   [Reproduced with permission. Source: Mirvis, S.E.; Young, J.W.R. Imaging in Trauma and Critical Care. Williams & Wilkins (Baltimore), 1992.]

distraction force (i.e., a force pulling along its length) is coupled with hyperextension of the neck. This results in bilateral C2 pedicle fractures with distraction of the anterior elements of the axis (joined to the atlas) from the posterior elements of C2. The spinal cord is severed at the C2 level, and death is instant.

An injury to the axis with the same fracture pattern has been observed in unrestrained individuals involved in high-velocity frontal crashes, with facial contact to the windshield. The distinction between judicial hanging and other causes of the hangman's fracture is an important one because the non-judicial hangman's fracture, unlike its judicial namesake, is generally not fatal. In fact, any neurological deficit associated with non-judicial hangman's fracture is usually temporary, and recovery following reduction and stabilization is usually complete. Spinal cord damage is probably minimized by: (1) the diameter of the spinal cord at the C2 level is less than one-half the diameter of the spinal canal (Steel 1968) (i.e., there is room to spare, even if the canal is somewhat compromised); (2) the fracture itself may enlarge rather than occlude the spinal canal (Harris 1996)—typically, the motor vehicle crash injury produces a separation of the anterior and posterior elements of the axis and a widening of the vertebral canal; and (3) the profound distractive force produced by judicial hanging is absent.

Two more formal terms that may be applied to bilateral pedicle fractures are "traumatic spondylolisthesis" and "traumatic spondylolysis." The term "spondylolisthesis" usually refers to bilateral pedicle fracture and an associated anterior vertebral displacement. The pars interarticularis may also be disrupted as the result of a congenital defect; therefore, the adjective "traumatic" is sometimes used to distinguish between the two. The term "spondylolysis" may be defined rather broadly as the dissolution or breaking up of a vertebra, but usually is used to refer specifically to a breaking of the pars interarticularis of the axis. Thus, the hangman's fracture may also be referred to as spondylolysis.

Spondylolisthesis may be graded based on the amount of forward displacement. Grade I involves displacement of <25% of the A-P dimension of the vertebral body; Grade II, between 25 and 50% displacement; Grade III, between 50 and 75% displacement; and Grade IV, >75% displacement (Oyesiku 1990).

Another method grades spondylolisthesis as Type I, II, or III (increasing severity), based on various characteristics of the injury. Type I traumatic spondylolisthesis is an isolated bilateral isthmus fracture (without the related injury of Types II or III). Type II, in addition to involving the bilateral fracture, is characterized by anterior disc compression and downward and forward angulation of the body of C2 (with respect to the body of C3). Type III is characterized by the bilateral isthmus fracture, disc disruption, and bilateral disruption of the facet joints. Although not included in the type definitions, a concomitant injury of traumatic spondylolisthesis is a wedge fracture of the subjacent vertebra, C3 (Effendi 1981; Levy 1986).

An injury mechanism has been attributed to each of the three types of traumatic spondylolisthesis: Type I—due to a combination of hyperextension plus compression; Type II—due to extension followed by flexion; and Type III—due to flexion followed by extension (Effendi 1981; Harris 1996).

Although relatively uncommon, the upper cervical spine may also be injured by lateral bending (lateral flexion). When it does occur, it typically produces ligament and muscle strain, contralateral to the direction of bending (Galli 1989). Lateral flexion more commonly occurs in conjunction with either vertical compression or rotation. The combination of lateral flexion and vertical compression produces the Jefferson fracture characteristic of compressive loading, but modified by the lateral bending so that the fragments of the Jefferson fracture are eccentrically (i.e., non-symmetrically) displaced. The combination of lateral flexion and rotation produces torticollis (Harris 1996), a twisting of the neck. Typically, torticollis results from relatively less violent head or neck motion (Harris 1996). The lateral flexion is somewhat self-limiting, in that the flexion is stopped when the head strikes the shoulder. Perhaps for this reason, there is little or no ligament disruption. This injury is considered stable. (As noted previously, lateral flexion may, in rare instances, produce a fracture of C2.)

Middle Cervical Region (C2–C5)

Compression Fractures

A characteristic fracture of the middle cervical spine region is the axial loading-type injuries that include compression-related fractures. Axial loading (i.e., along the length of the spine) of an erect vertebral column produces a characteristic fracture called a compression fracture or burst fracture. Essentially, bursting is a comminuted fracture of the vertebral body. It tends to occur when a compressive load is applied to a pre-straightened spine (Harris 1996); hence, it is a good example of the importance of initial position (i.e., neck position at the time the force is applied) on injury occurrence. This loading is most typically via contact loading to the top of the head or to the buttocks (via an upward [i.e., cephalically directed] force). One way a compression fracture may occur in the vehicular crash environment is in conjunction with vehicle rollover, which can produce axial loading, as illustrated in the following case study:

Case Study. The subject vehicle, a 1986 pickup truck, was involved in a single-vehicle rollover accident. According to the driver, he was experiencing hallucinations and suddenly swerved to avoid a large, imaginary object that he perceived to be crossing in front of him. The rollover produced moderate roof crush (Figure 3.19), and the occupant received a diving-type injury due to the inertia of the torso when the vehicle was inverted (similar to the injury produced by a swimmer diving into shallow water). The CT of C5 (Figure 3.20) shows the vertical body fracture, typical of burst fractures, and also shows a laminar fracture. Thus, the vertebra was essentially broken into two halves. Note that although the two halves are shown fairly well aligned in the CT (i.e., they do not appear to be intruding into the space occupied by the cord), they may have been briefly displaced during the crash and moved back in place when the CT was taken. The injury produced quadriplegia at C5.

When an axial force is applied to the spine, much of the force is converted into deformation of the intervertebral discs. If a disc undergoes sufficient

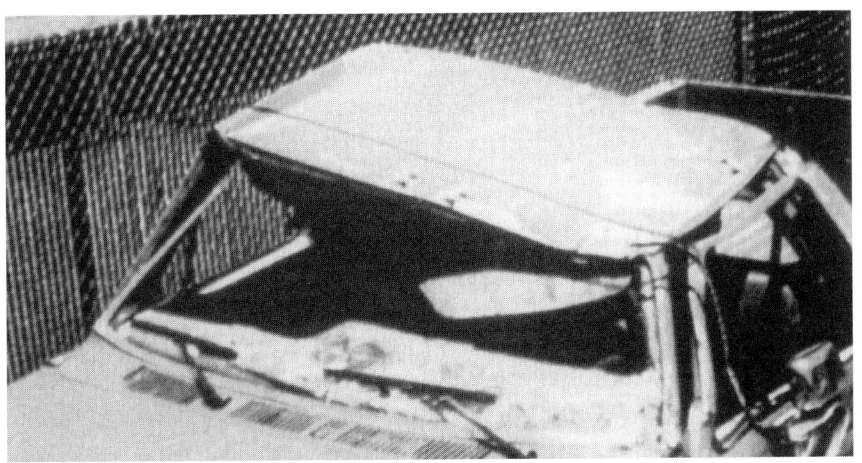

Figure 3.19 Case Study III—Subject vehicle.

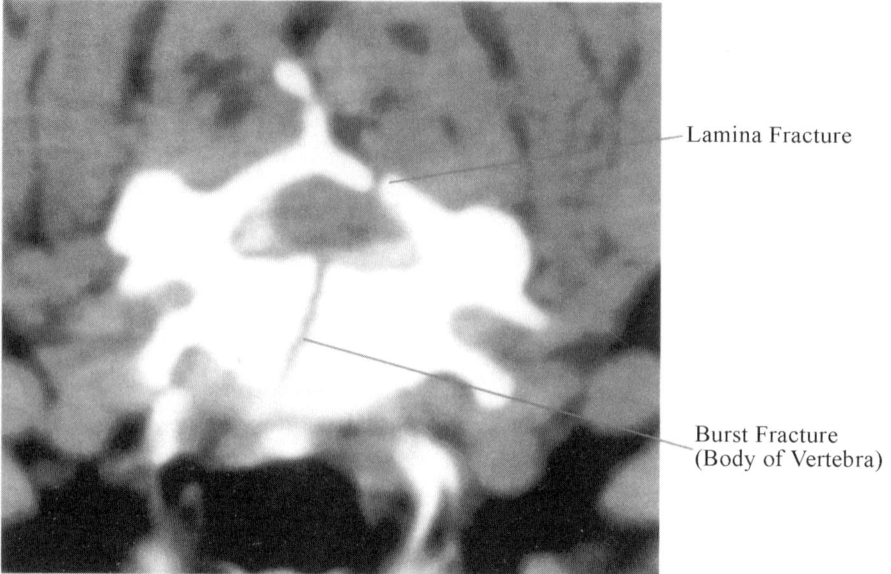

Figure 3.20   Case Study III—Burst fracture (CT).

compression, the intra-discal pressure will extrude the gelatinous "filling" of the nucleus pulposus through the end plate of an adjacent vertebral body (usually the one above the disc). This, in turn, causes the vertebral body to explode, producing a comminuted (multiple fragments) vertebral body fracture. The fracture may vary from one with relatively few fragments and relatively little dispersion to one with many fragments and some fragments widely displaced.

Note that a vertebral body with a burst fracture might appear in a lateral view radiograph very similar to a vertebral body with a flexion teardrop fracture (e.g., compare the burst fracture in Figure 3.21 with the teardrop fracture in Figure 3.22). However, a burst fracture does not generally affect other parts of the vertebrae, and thus the absence of flexion characteristics, such as fanning out of the posterior processes, helps to distinguish between flexion and burst injuries on the lateral view. Also, an additional view may be used to help distinguish between the two. For example, in frontal view, the burst fracture (unlike the teardrop fracture), frequently displays a vertical fracture line, extending the full S-I dimension of the affected vertebral body.

The burst fracture fragments of the vertebral body may be dispersed in all directions, but retropulsion of fragments of the posterior vertebral body is

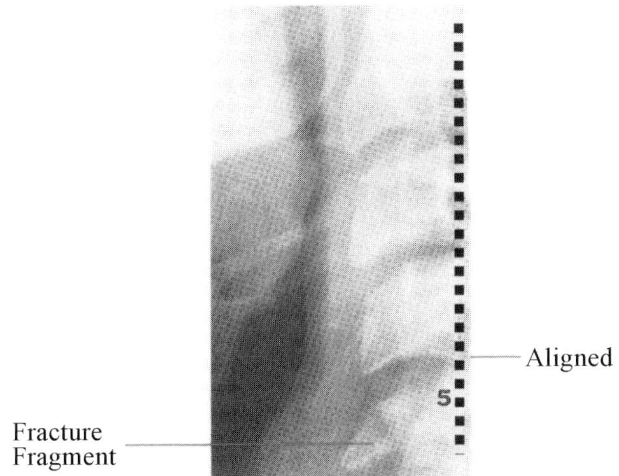

Figure 3.21 Burst fracture (lateral view). [Reproduced with permission. Source: Harris, J.; Mirvis, S. Radiology of Acute Cervical Spine Trauma, 3rd Edition. Williams & Wilkins (Baltimore), 1996.]

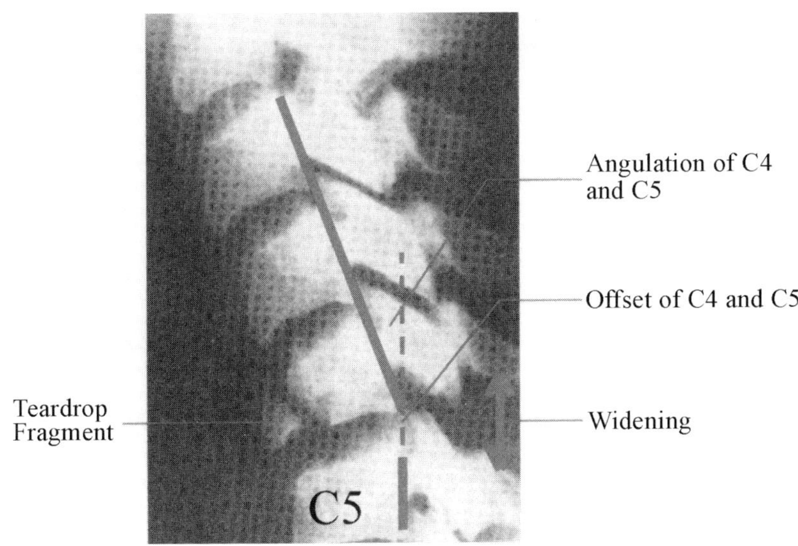

Figure 3.22 Teardrop fracture (lateral view). [Reproduced with permission. Source: Harris, J.; Mirvis, S. Radiology of Acute Cervical Spine Trauma, 3rd Edition. Williams & Wilkins (Baltimore), 1996.]

most typical. This is the type of fragmentation that may impinge upon and consequently injure the spinal cord. Newer imaging methods have indicated that a burst fracture is frequently accompanied by fracture of one or both laminae (Harris 1996) (Figure 3.20). In this scenario, depending on the severity of the bone fragmentation, the injury could be considered either stable or unstable (that is, it may or may not have the potential for subsequent neurological injury, even without any additional external trauma). However, if bilateral laminar fracture accompanies the vertebral body fracture, the injury is considered unstable even though the posterior ligamentous complex, including the facet joints, may be intact (Harris 1996).

Trauma to the mid-cervical region may also occur in the vehicular crash environment from extension movements of the neck. This can happen typically in a rear impact, if the torso is pushed forward with respect to the head (so that, in effect, the head moves backward with respect to the torso). It can also happen during a frontal crash, if the forehead of an unbelted occupant impacts and then stays in contact with the sun visor, while the torso continues some forward and upward movement. As is the case with flexion injuries, extension injuries are dependent on a variety of factors, including the direction and magnitude of the force causing the extension.

The extension teardrop fracture is similar to the flexion teardrop fracture, in that the latter is also named after an avulsion fracture of the anterior inferior corner of the vertebral body. This part of the vertebral body is the attachment point for the anterior longitudinal ligament, which is thought to avulse the fragment during neck extension (Harris 1996). Because of the disruption of the anterior longitudinal ligament, the extension teardrop fracture is considered unstable, but only in extension. The posterior ligamentous complex generally is not disrupted by this injury; therefore, the extension teardrop fracture is considered stable in flexion. Extension teardrop fractures typically occur in older individuals or others with degenerative disease of the spine (Boden 1991).

Hyperextension Dislocation

If there is a sufficiently large posterior displacement associated with extension movement, both the anterior longitudinal ligament and the intervertebral disc may be disrupted. The anterior longitudinal ligament will tear and, if the extension is sufficient, will eventually rupture completely. The intervertebral disc may tear more or less in half, in a horizontal plane, or may remain essentially intact but be torn away from the inferior end plate of the suprajacent vertebra. The strong Sharpe's fibers, which form the outer covering of the annulus fibrosis of the intervertebral disc, may tear off the front part of the bottom of the vertebral body, thereby creating an avulsion fracture of the anterior aspect of the inferior end plate. Although the hyperextension dislocation avulsion fracture may appear similar to an extension teardrop fracture, the hyperextension dislocation typically does not involve the upper cervical spine, whereas the extension teardrop typically is limited to C2. Also, the extension teardrop typically involves an osteoporotic vertebra. The fracture fragments produced by the two types of fracture are often distinguishable by shape: the hyperextension dislocation avulsion fragment is wider than it is high (i.e., is greater in anterior-posterior dimension than in superior-inferior dimension), whereas the reverse is generally true for the extension teardrop fragment (Harris 1996).

If the posterior vertebral displacement is sufficient, the posterior longitudinal ligament may be torn from the subjacent vertebral body. (The ligament, however, may remain intact.) The posterior displacement of the dislocated vertebra will also narrow the space in the vertebral canal until the spinal cord is compressed between the posterior aspect of the vertebral body (anteriorly) and the ligamentum flavum or the vertebral lamina (posteriorly) (Baxt 1985; Rosen 1988). As mentioned previously, this simultaneous compression of the anterior and posterior surfaces of the spinal cord produces neither an anterior cord syndrome nor a posterior cord syndrome but, perhaps counterintuitively, a central cord syndrome (Rosen 1988). Additional insight into this injury mechanism can be obtained by noting that a hyperextension dislocation is often accompanied by facial bruising or facial bone fracture (Harris 1996). Thus, hyperextension dislocation is frequently associated with impact to the face or forehead.

Note that for individuals with preexisting spinal degeneration (e.g., osteophytes), relatively mild trauma may produce a central cord syndrome but with a slightly different injury mechanism. The cord is still compressed posteriorly by the in-bulging ligamentum flavum; but anteriorly, rather than being compressed by the posterior aspect of the vertebral body proper, the spinal cord is compressed by osteophytes projecting posteriorly from the vertebral body (Adams 1983; Baxt 1985). This compressive mechanism is relatively common among the elderly (Barr 1988; Boden 1991) and is sometimes referred to as the Taylor mechanism.

Apparently, these hyperextension dislocations are within the elastic limits of the facet joint capsules and the other posterior ligaments, because even though both the anterior longitudinal ligament and the posterior longitudinal ligament may be disrupted, the displaced vertebra reduces spontaneously. That is, the still-intact ligaments and muscles combine to pull the vertebra back into place (Baxt 1985; Pike 1990).

Extension with Rotation

In the vehicular crash environment, the combination of extension and rotation can occur in several different ways, including an off-center crash, a two-stage crash, or a crash with an out-of-position occupant. The off-center crash refers to the scenario where the subject vehicle is struck off-center from the rear, so that the occupant both has his head pushed backward and rotated. The two-stage crash refers to the subject vehicle being struck twice, perhaps by one vehicle, which spins the car around (thereby causing the head to rotate), followed by impact with a second vehicle (or object, such as a tree), which contacts the vehicle squarely in the rear, thereby causing neck extension. In a crash with an out-of-position occupant, the out-of-position occupant could have his head turned to the side (e.g., to look at something on the roadside or talk to another occupant) at the time the vehicle is rear ended, thereby adding neck extension to an already existing neck rotation.

The unilateral comminuted facet fracture (Figure 3.23) is also referred to as a hyperextension fracture dislocation. Typically, the head is rotated posteriorly and inferiorly (i.e., as if looking back and down over the shoulder). As a result, the anterior longitudinal ligament is disrupted, and the facet joint contralateral to the direction of motion is fractured and impacted (i.e., margins of fracture driven into each other). The fracture is usually quite extensive, and the facets may be severely comminuted, if not completely obliterated. The forces are such that the suprajacent vertebra translates anteriorly. The amount of anterior translation associated with this injury is typically larger than the anterior translation associated with anterior subluxation (3–6 mm versus <3 mm) (0.12–0.24 in. versus <0.12 in.). The unilateral facet fracture may be accompanied by lamina and/or spinous process fractures (Harris 1996).

The posterior rotation also causes the contralateral facet to disrupt (but not generally to fracture). The combination of the facet fracture on the side contralateral to the direction of rotation, and facet disruption (partial or complete dislocation) ipsilateral to the direction of rotation, allows the anterior translation that characterizes this injury. Both facets are disrupted; therefore, the injury is considered unstable.

The unilateral comminuted facet fracture is distinguished from the unilateral facet dislocation, which can be due to a combination of rotation and

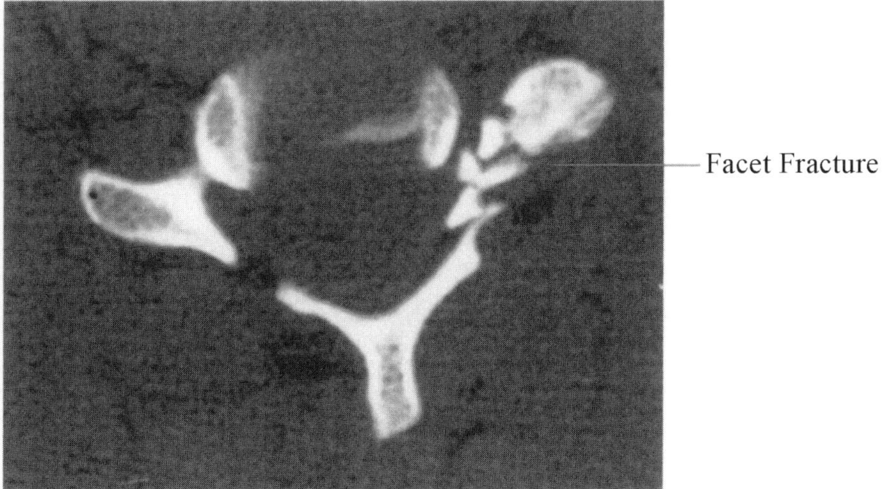

Figure 3.23   Unilateral facet fracture (comminuted) (CT).

flexion, and which does not involve comminuted fracture of the facet. This distinction provides a good example of how information regarding injury mechanism may provide guidance regarding treatment. Anterior displacement is typically associated with flexion, for which traction in extension might be a suitable treatment. If the anterior displacement is associated with extension (e.g., a hyperextension rotation fracture dislocation), then if it is treated with traction in extension, the "treatment' would be replicating, at least in part, the injury-producing motion (Harris 1996) and hence might not be desirable.

Pillar Fracture

The pillar fracture occurs generally when the combination of extension and rotation compresses the articular pillar (inter-facet articulating masses) between the suprajacent and subjacent pillars. Under such conditions, a pillar fracture is produced ipsilateral to the direction of rotation (i.e., if the neck movement is such that the nose moves to the right, the right pillar is fractured). The fracture is usually vertical or nearly vertical, with little or no comminution. When comminuted, the fragment is usually displaced posteriorly. This posterior displacement is made evident on a lateral view plain film: the posterior cortical margins of the left and right pillars do not line up, i.e., are not superimposed and thus appear as two separate lines (Figure 3.24). Note

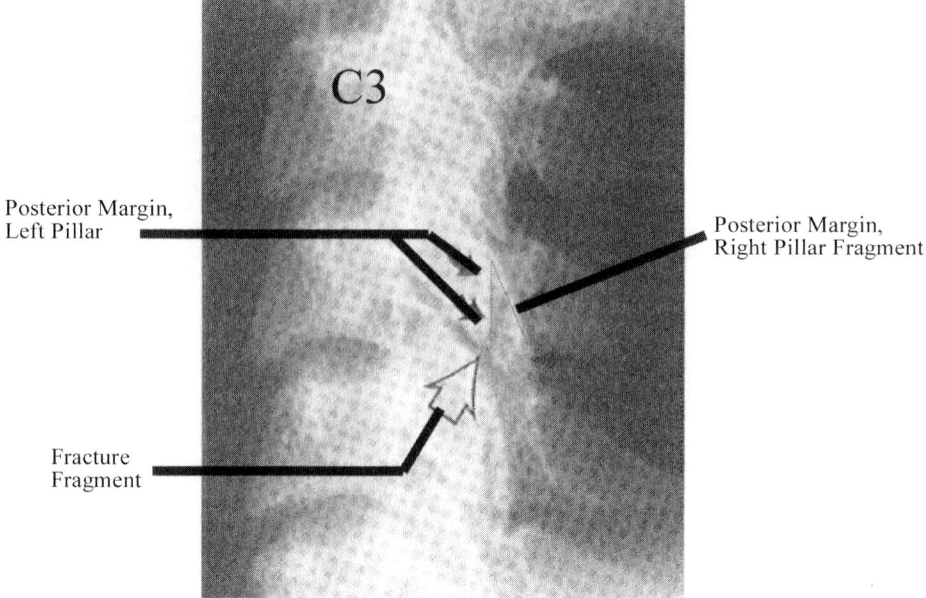

Figure 3.24 Pillar fracture (lateral view). [Reproduced with permission. Source: Harris, J.; Mirvis, S. Radiology of Acute Cervical Spine Trauma, 3rd Edition. Williams & Wilkins (Baltimore), 1996.]

that the pillar fracture is distinguished from the unilateral comminuted facet fracture, in that the unilateral comminuted facet fracture is located contralaterally with respect to the direction of rotation and is a severely comminuted fracture.

Anterior Subluxation

(Note: Subluxation is synonymous with partial dislocation. Thus, in the remainder of this discussion, a subluxation is sometimes referred to as a partial dislocation. Although subluxations can occur at any level of the cervical spine, they are most common in the mid-cervical spine.)

Anterior subluxation (also called anterolisthesis) refers to the forward displacement of one vertebral body with respect to an adjacent vertebral body—either the one immediately above (the suprajacent vertebra), or the one immediately below (the subjacent vertebra). Anterior subluxation is frequently a flexion injury. When caused by flexion, the anterior subluxation may occur either alone or in conjunction with other flexion-related injuries.

As discussed in Chapter 1, the two- or three-column concept of vertebral structure leads one to expect that any pivoting movement of the anterior of a vertebra will have a reciprocal pivoting movement of the posterior of the vertebra. The "anterior" aspects of the anterior subluxation include a downward angulation of the anterior vertebral body and/or a forward translation of the vertebral body with respect to the body of the subjacent vertebra. Note that this translation is rather minimal, typically being in the range of 1–3 mm (0.04–0.12 in.) (Holdsworth 1970). The anterior longitudinal ligament remains intact, as does the anterior portion of the intervertebral disc, but the disc space may be narrowed anteriorly. The "posterior" aspects of the anterior subluxation may include disruption of the posterior ligamentous complex, including the posterior longitudinal ligament, the interspinous ligament, the ligamentum flavum, and the facet joint capsules (Holdsworth 1970; Harris 1996).

The posterior ligament disruption may also present as widening of the posterior region of the disc space, displacement of inferior articulating facets with respect to subjacent facets, and widening of interspinous or interlaminal space (fanning). The fanning is somewhat analogous to the opening of a bellows: the front of the bellows moves closer together, and the handles of the bellows move farther apart. These may all be observed on Figure 3.25. If ligaments undergo minor stretching, they may be described as being "sprained." Therefore, a sprain associated with flexion may be specified as a hyperflexion sprain. If ligaments are stretched to the point of significant tearing (or even rupturing), such an injury may then be labeled as a severe sprain.

Anterior subluxation is primarily a flexion injury; thus, the radiographic signs of anterior subluxation are accentuated in flexion and mitigated in extension. Therefore, a lateral radiograph of the neck in flexion (to the extent that flexion is possible) may be included to supplement the normal position radiograph. (This is an example of how knowledge of injury mechanism can be useful in diagnosing injury.)

As already mentioned, when an anterior subluxation occurs, the anterior longitudinal ligament and the anterior portion of the intervertebral disc remain intact; therefore, an anterior subluxation typically is stable (at least initially). However, anterior subluxations have a relatively high incidence of inadequate ligament healing and subsequent development into an unstable injury (which may then lead to neurological injury). Estimates of the incidence of delayed

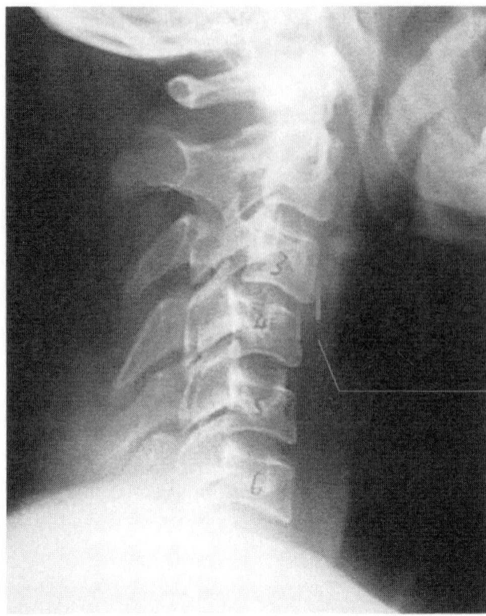

Figure 3.25 Anterior subluxation of C3 on C4.

instability following anterior subluxation range from approximately one in five to as high as one in two (Cheshire 1969).

Wedge Fracture

When a vertebra is fractured as a result of flexion, one or both of the adjacent vertebrae causing the subject vertebra to fracture may compress the anterior region of the vertebral body. As a result, the lateral view of the vertebral body appears somewhat like a wedge (Figure 3.26), hence the name "wedge fracture." The interspinous, supraspinous, and nuchal ligaments may be disrupted in conjunction with this fracture, but the other ligaments generally remain intact; thus, the wedge fracture is stable (at least initially). If the original injury does include disruption of the posterior ligamentous complex and the ligaments do not heal properly, the result could be an unstable spine. In this instance, the wedge fracture may lead to late-developing (additional) neurological injury. The wedge fracture often displays other characteristics in the lateral view, in addition to the shape of the fracture. These include buckling of the anterior cortex and disruption of the superior end plate of the vertebral body (Harris 1996).

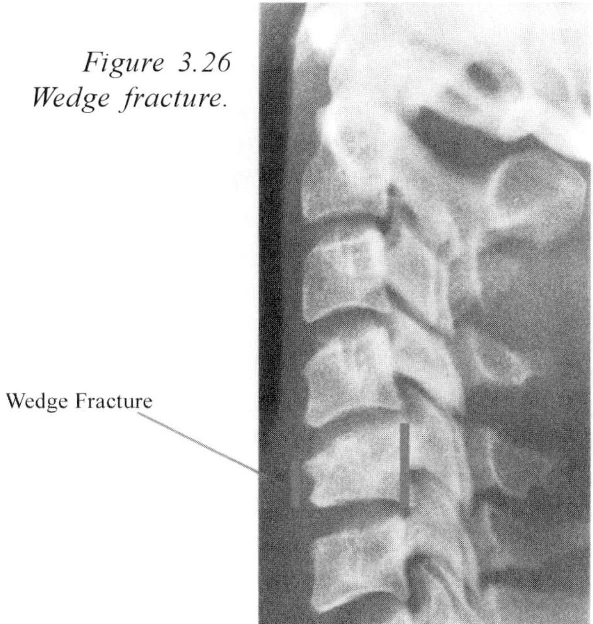

Figure 3.26
Wedge fracture.

Teardrop Fracture (Flexion)

The term "teardrop fracture" refers to a characteristic fragment that breaks off from the anteroinferior corner of the vertebral body. The fragment usually is roughly triangular in shape and apparently reminded the nomenclaturist of the shape of a tear.

This teardrop fracture is often associated with relatively violent neck motion, and it has a high incidence of spinal cord injury associated with it. In general, the teardrop fragment does not impinge on the cord and cause cord injury; rather, the occurrence of the teardrop fragment serves as a "marker" that cord injury is likely. Concomitant injury includes disruption of both the anterior and posterior ligament complexes, including bilateral subluxation or complete dislocation of the facet joints.

The flexion teardrop fracture is unstable, and, as mentioned previously, neurological injury is common. Typically, the fractured vertebra is displaced posteriorly and rotated anteriorly (Figure 3.22), and angulation of the vertebral column results. The spinal canal is thereby compromised (Figure 3.27). Usually, the frontal region of the spinal cord is injured, and this produces the anterior cord syndrome.

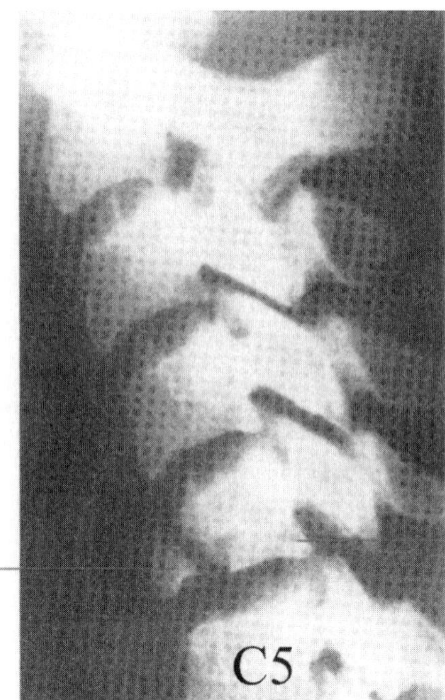

Figure 3.27 Teardrop fracture (flexion). [Reproduced with permission. Source: Harris, J.; Mirvis, S. Radiology of Acute Cervical Spine Trauma, 3rd Edition. Williams & Wilkins (Baltimore), 1996.]

As with other flexion injuries that disrupt the posterior ligamentous complex, teardrop fractures are characterized by a bellows-like spreading of the spinous processes (Figure 3.22). The teardrop fracture may also be associated with neurological damage via another mechanism, involving a concomitant injury; the posterior of the vertebral body often fractures as well, and this posterior fragment may be displaced posteriorly (retropulsed) into the spinal canal (Helms 1989).

The following is an example of one way a flexion teardrop fracture may be produced in the vehicular crash environment:

Case Study. The subject vehicle fell backward off of an elevated highway, landing on the rear of the vehicle. As far as the vehicle occupants were concerned, it was essentially a high-speed rear impact (Figure 3.28). The right front seat occupant had his seat fully reclined (nearly horizontal) and was not belted. Upon impact, he slid along the seat back into the rear seat, at which point his flexed neck received compressive loading when his head impacted the seat back

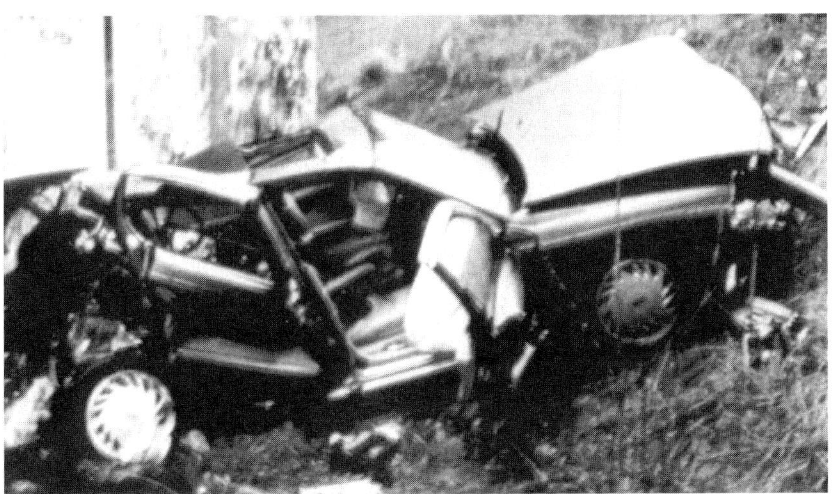

Figure 3.28   Case Study IV—Subject vehicle exterior.

of the rear seat. This produced a variety of injuries, including ligament injuries, which permitted vertebral displacement, which in turn
produced severe spinal cord compression (Figures 3.29 and 3.30).
The patient became a quadriplegic. (It is noted by comparison that
the driver, who was belted and whose seat was not fully reclined,
was virtually uninjured and was able to extricate himself from the
vehicle and go to get help.)

Lower Cervical Region (C5-T1)

Spinous Process Fracture

The spinous processes serve as attachment points for various muscles (e.g.,
trapezius, rhomboid). These muscles may be referred to as the neck exten-
sors. Basically, they are located in the posterior and posterolateral regions of
the neck. When they contract, they produce neck extension and also help to
"protect" against excessive neck flexion. When these muscles contract suddenly and/or forcefully, the pull on the spinous process may be sufficient to
fracture the process. This fracture often occurs close to where the process
joins the rest of the vertebra (Orrison 1989) (Figure 3.31).

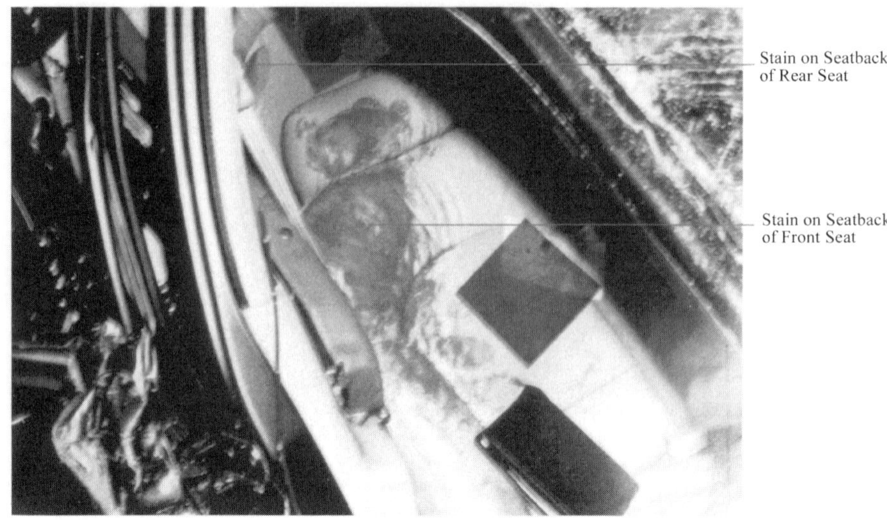

Figure 3.29   Case Study IV—Subject vehicle interior.

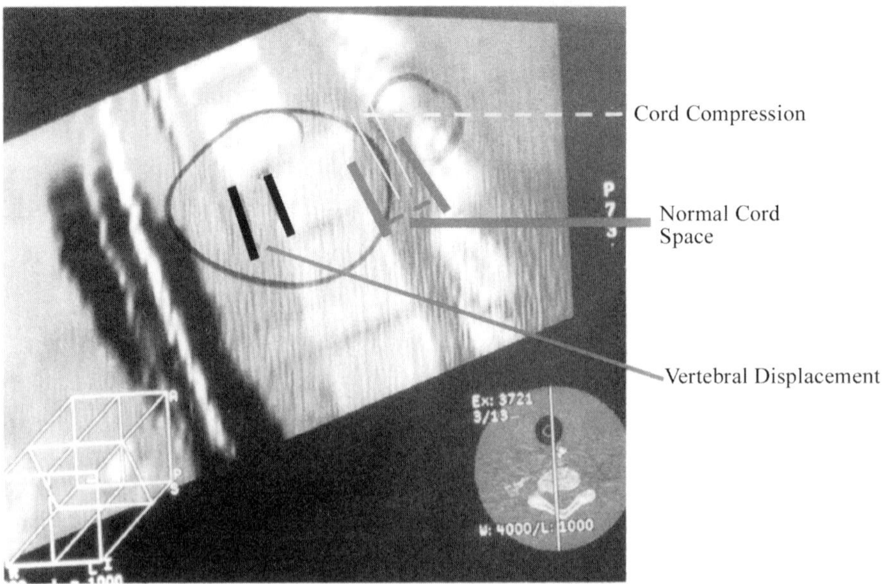

Figure 3.30   Case Study IV—Vertebral displacement and spinal cord compression.

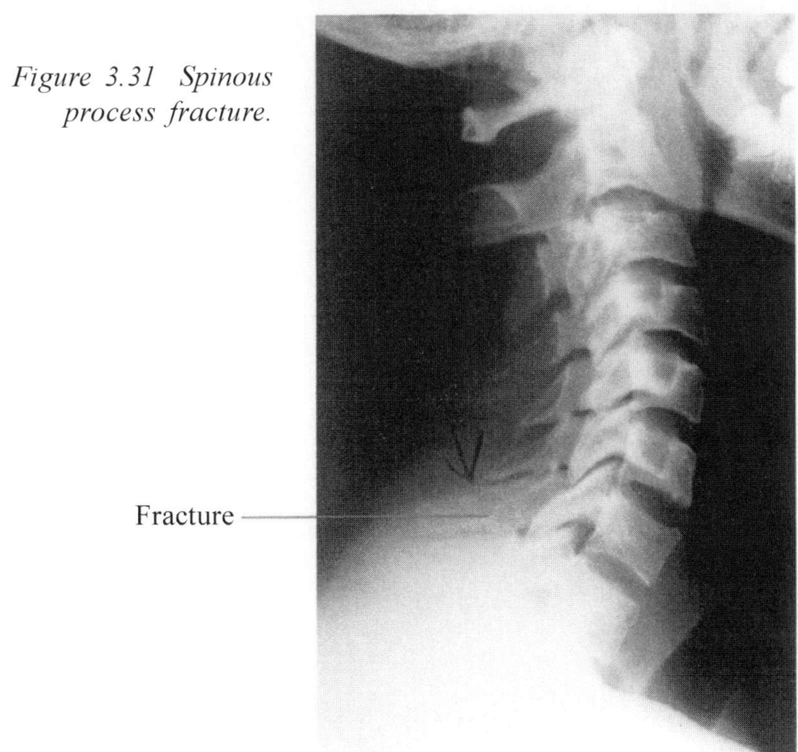

Figure 3.31 Spinous process fracture.

Most frequently, spinous process fracture will occur at C6 or C7 (Orrison 1989). Perhaps not unrelated, these are the two most prominent cervical spinous processes (White 1990). With this type of injury, ligament disruption is minimal, and the fracture is usually stable (Levy 1986). In rare instances, the fracture extends to the lamina of the vertebra, in which case a laminar fragment could impinge on the spinal cord and thereby cause neurological injury.

Apparently, spinous process fracture was observed historically in men who shoveled heavy, moist clay; thus, this injury may still be referred to as clay shoveler's fracture. Note that spinous process fracture may also occur from extension and indeed, the same eponym, clay shoveler's fracture, may be used. It would then refer to a hyperextension process fracture due to an entirely different mechanism, namely, the forceful contact between the spinous processes of two adjacent vertebrae.

Bilateral Facet Dislocation

Bilateral facet dislocation is due to a relatively "pure" flexion, with little or no rotational component. (There is, of course, rotation of the head in the mid-sagittal plane associated with flexion, but there is minimal rotation of the head about the longitudinal axis of the neck.) As in the case of anterior subluxation, the flexion results in disruption of the posterior ligamentous complex (posterior longitudinal ligament, interspinous ligament, nuchal ligament, posterior annulus fibrosis of disc), but disruption of the anterior ligamentous complex and tearing of the intervertebral disc occurs as well. Thus, the affected vertebrae are relatively free to move with respect to each other, and a vertebra may move forward and upward with respect to its subjacent vertebra, until the inferior facet of the disrupted facet joint becomes nestled above and slightly forward of the superior facet. Both the right and left facets move in a similar manner; thus, this type of injury is referred to as bilateral facet dislocation (Figure 3.32). If the injury causes the vertebra to move forward only enough so that the facets rest on top of each other, it is referred to as "perched" facets (Figure 3.33).

The formation resulting from bilateral facet dislocation is sometimes referred to as locked facets. If the facets were somehow bound in this position,

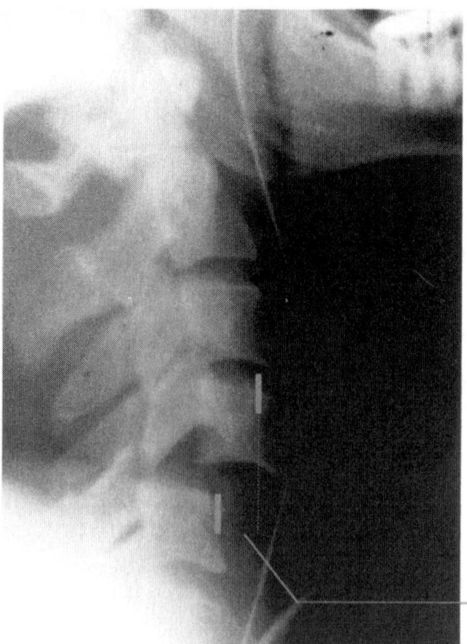

Figure 3.32 Bilateral facet dislocation (lateral view).

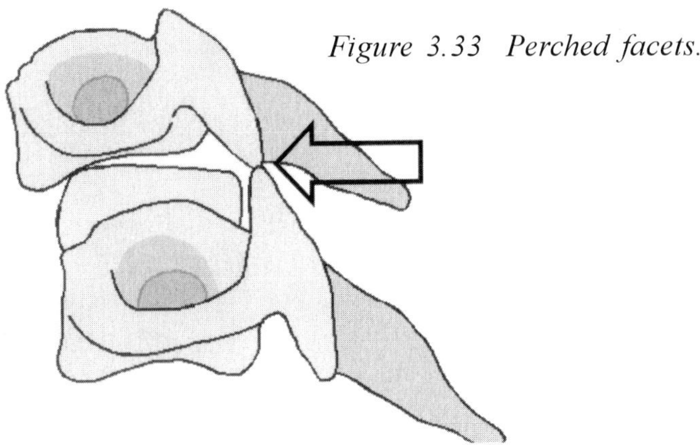

Figure 3.33   Perched facets.

they would indeed be locked. However, they often are not. Quite the contrary, this injury frequently is very unstable; the facets are prone to move, and the spinal cord is susceptible to injury from this subsequent movement. Indeed, bilateral facet dislocations are associated with a high incidence of neurological (spinal cord) injury (Yoganandan 1990). Thus, it may be more appropriate to refer to this injury as bilateral facet dislocation or to use some other terminology that does not run the risk of inadvertently portraying this as a stable and, in that sense, a self-limiting injury.

Bilateral facet dislocations most frequently occur at C5 to C7. This is the region of the cervical spine where the canal is relatively narrow, and hence where the cervical spinal cord is relatively susceptible to compressive injury (Galli 1989). The bilateral facet dislocation shown in Figure 3.32 produced complete quadriplegia.

Bilateral facet dislocations are considered mechanically unstable (Baxt 1985; Rhea 1988). If only one facet joint (right or left) is dislocated and comes to rest in the inferior portion of the intervertebral foramen, that facet is indeed "locked" (due at least in part to the forces exerted on it by the ipsilateral, intact facet). Thus, the terminology "unilateral locked facet" is quite appropriate (Figure 3.34). The mechanism of unilateral facet dislocation (unilateral locked facet) is discussed in the next section.

Bilateral facet dislocation is frequently associated with a facet fracture (Levy 1986). A bilateral facet (complete) dislocation typically is associated with anterior displacement of at least 50% of the A-P dimension of the vertebral body (Figure 3.35). Note: By contrast, the unilateral facet dislocation (Figure 3.36) typically is associated with <50% anterior displacement.

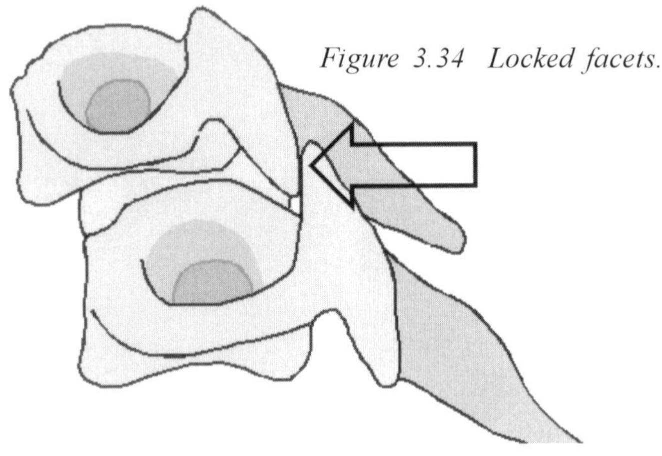

Figure 3.34   Locked facets.

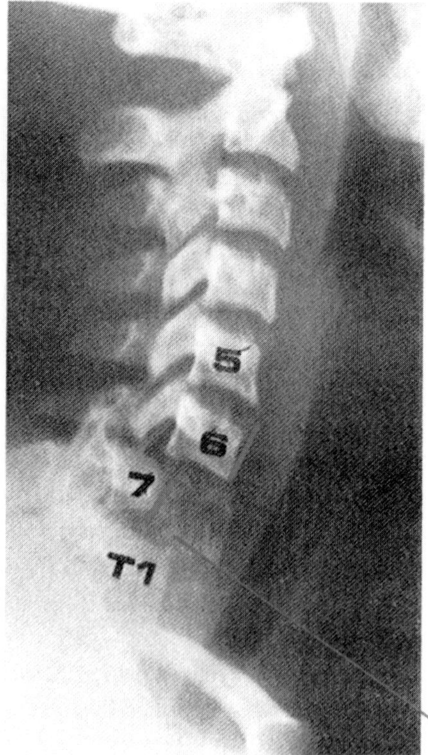

Offset (>50%)

Figure 3.35   Bilateral facet dislocation.   [Reproduced with permission.   Source: Rockwood, C.A., Jr.; Green, D.P.; Bucholz, R.W. Rockwood and Green's Fractures in Adults, 3rd Edition. Lippincott (Philadelphia), 1991.]

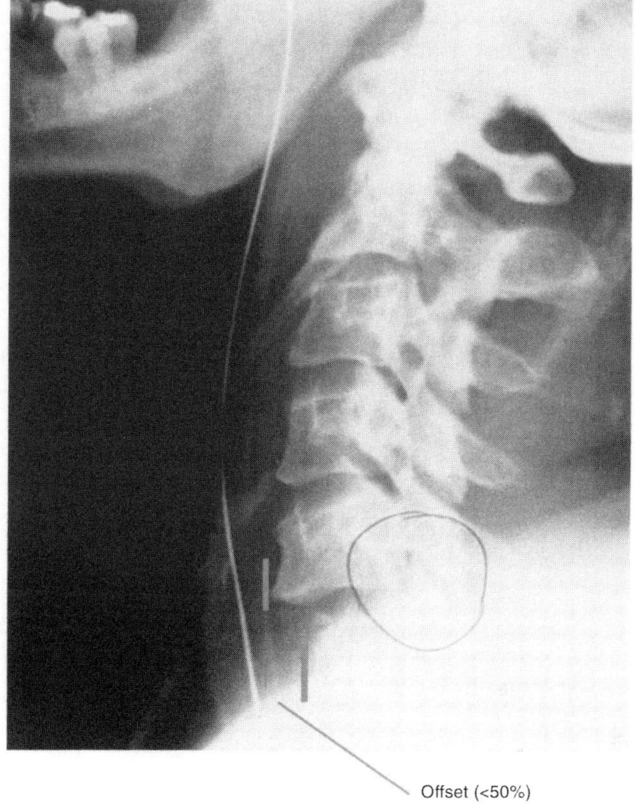

Figure 3.36   Unilateral facet dislocation.

Flexion with Rotation

When cervical spine injury results from the combination of neck flexion and rotation, the injury is usually unilateral facet dislocation (Figure 3.36); that is, the facet joint contralateral to the direction of motion is dislocated. Thus, if the head rotates such that the nose moves to the right, the right side facet joint acts as a pivot and the left facet joint is disrupted. The upper facet and the associated articular mass of the left facet joint move anteriorly and superiorly until the facet becomes lodged in the intervertebral foramen, that is, between the lower facet (more precisely, the subjacent articular mass) and the vertebral body. The dislocated facet will tend to remain in that position, even during subsequent neck movement, and thus may be referred to as a locked facet.

Although the dislocated and locked facet is the signature of a flexion-with-rotation injury, other associated injuries are quite common. The posterior ligamentous complex, including the posterior part of the intervertebral disc, is usually disrupted; hence, the injury also is characterized by increased interspinous and interlaminal distance (bellows or fanning). Also, either of the facets associated with the dislocated joint may fracture. If this occurs, the resulting fracture fragment may pose a risk to the spinal cord; hence, the injury would then be considered more severe and be treated accordingly (Harris 1993). The capsule of the contralateral facet (the facet that serves as the pivot) may also be disrupted.

Injuries Subsequent to Preexisting Conditions

An individual with preexisting pathology involving the cervical spine is at greater risk for sustaining injury to the neck in a motor vehicle crash. Any condition resulting in compromise of the structural integrity of the spine, such as osteoporosis or arthritis, increases the risk of trauma to the bone and soft tissue structures in the neck. Furthermore, congenital or chronic narrowing of the spinal canal (spinal stenosis) as seen in cervical spondylosis, predisposes the person to associated spinal cord injury in the event of a neck injury. The following case underlines this point:

> **Case Study.** A 37-year-old lap-and-shoulder-belt-restrained female driving a 1989 full-size car was negotiating a left turn at an intersection when her vehicle was struck by a 1986 luxury-size car traveling in the opposite direction. The low-speed impact was to the right front fender of her vehicle and produced a force coming from "2 o'clock." Upon EMS arrival at the scene, the woman was found walking around and appeared to be uninjured (with the exception of small abrasions). The damage to the vehicles was noted to be minor. Based on these observations, the EMS personnel elected not to transport the woman to a trauma center. However, she began to complain of burning and tingling in her hands. This alerted the rescue crew to a possible spinal cord injury. She was subsequently transported to the trauma center. The patient was diagnosed with central cord syndrome, based on clinical presentation. This is a condition in which the spinal cord is compressed with resultant injury to the central aspect of the cord at a particular level. Due to the neural organization of the spinal cord, upper extremity sensation and function is affected with sparing of the

lower extremities. This particular patient presented with burning and tingling as well as paresthesis in her hands. Plain film, CT, and MR imaging of her cervical spine revealed severe stenosis and osteophyte formation in the lower cervical spine, as well as slight anterolisthesis of C5 on C6. These findings are consistent with hyperflexion of a cervical spine that had chronic degenerative changes (Figure 3.37).

In summary, we have discussed elements of the anatomy and physiology of the neck and spine, the images used in the initial assessment of trauma, the injuries encountered, and the injury mechanisms associated with them. We hope that this material will provide members of the interdisciplinary automotive safety community with information that will help them to provide additional benefit to the motoring public and to the population at large.

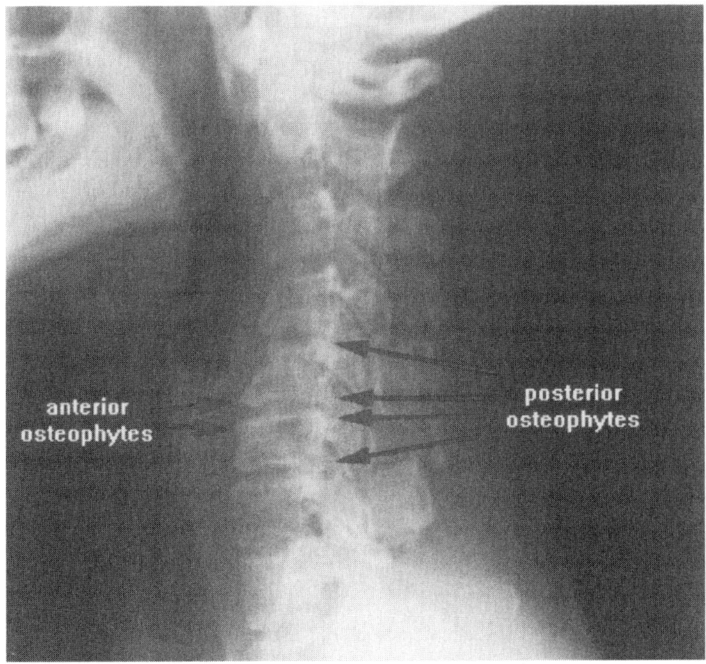

Figure 3.37   Case Study V—Preexisting spinal degeneration.

References

Adams, J. (1983). *Outline of Fractures*. Churchill Livingstone (Edinburgh).

Allen, Jr., B. (1989). "Fractures and Dislocations," in Sherk, H.H. (ed.), *The Cervical Spine*. The Cervical Spine Research Society, Lippincott (Philadelphia), 286–298.

Allen, Jr., B.; Ferguson, R.; Lehrnann, T.; et al. (1982). "Mechanistic Classification of Closed Indirect Fractures and Dislocations of the Lower Cervical Spine." *Spine* 7:1–27.

Anderson, L.; Clark, C. (1989). "Fractures of the Odontoid Process of the Axis," in Sherk, H.H. (ed.), *The Cervical Spine,* 2nd Edition. The Cervical Spine Research Society, Lippincott (Philadelphia), 325–341.

Anderson, L.; D'Alonzo, R. (1974). "Fractures of the Odontoid Process of the Axis." *J. Bone Joint Surg.* 56A:1663.

Barr, J. (1988). "The Treatment of Spinal Trauma," in Burke, J.; Boyd, R.; McCabe, C., Trauma Management Yearbook (Chicago), 512–532.

Baxt, W. (1985). *Trauma: The First Hour*. Appleton-Century-Crofts (Norwalk).

Benson, D.; Anderson, D. (1988). "Fractures, Dislocations, Infections and Tumors of Atlas and Axis," in Chapman, M.; Madison, M., *Operative Orthopaedics*. Lippincott (Philadelphia), 3:1883–1892.

Bland, J.H. (1994). *Disorders of the Cervical Spine: Diagnosis and Medical Management,* 2nd Edition. Saunders (Philadelphia).

Boden, S.D.; Wiesel, S.W.; Laws, Jr., E.R. (1991). *The Aging Spine: Essentials of Pathophysiology, Diagnosis and Treatment*. Saunders (Philadelphia).

Bohlman, H.H. (1986). "The Neck," Chap. 6 in D'Ambrosia, R.D. (ed.), *Musculoskeletal Disorders*, 2nd Edition. Lippincott (Philadelphia), 219–286.

Bontrager, K.L. (1993). *Textbook of Radiographic Positioning and Related Anatomy*, 3rd Edition. Mosby Year Book (St. Louis).

Bushong, S.C. (1988). *Magnetic Resonance Imaging: Physical and Biological Principles*. Mosby (St. Louis).

Byrne, T.N.; Waxman, S.G. (1990). *Spinal Cord Compression*. F.A. Davis (Philadelphia).

Camins, M.B.; O'Leary, P.F. (eds.) (1992). *Disorders of the Cervical Spine*. Williams & Wilkins (Baltimore).

Campbell, W.H.; Cantrill, S.V. (1988). "Neck Injuries," Chap. 21 in Rosen, P.; Baker, F.J.; Barkin, R.M.; Braen, G.R.; Dailey, R.H.; Levy, R.C. (eds.), *Emergency Medicine: Concepts and Clinical Practice*, 2nd Edition, Vol. 1 (Trauma). Mosby (St. Louis), 419–430.

Carroll, C.N.; McAfee, P. (1988), "Fractures and Dislocations of Cervical 3–7," Chap. 150 in Chapman, M.W. (ed.), *Operative Orthopaedics*. Lippincott (Philadelphia), 1893–1904.

Chandler, D.; Kropf, M.; Waters, R. (1992). "Classification of Lower Cervical Spine Injuries," in Camins M.; O'Leary, P., *Disorders of the Cervical Spine*. Williams & Wilkins (Baltimore), 628.

Cheshire, D.J. (1969). "The Stability of the Cervical Spine Following the Conservative Treatment of Fractures and Fracture-Dislocations," *Paraplegia* 7(3):193–203.

Clemente, C.D. (ed.) (1985). *Anatomy of the Human Body, by Henry Gray*, 30th Edition (American Edition). Lea & Febiger (Philadelphia).

Clintron, E.; Gilula, L.; Murphy, W.; et al. (1981). "Widened Disc Space: Sign of Cervical Hyperextension Injury," *Radiol.* 141:639–644.

Connolly, J.F. (1988). *Fracture Complications.* Year Book Medical Publishers (Chicago).

Daffner, R.H. (1996). *Imaging of Vertebral Trauma,* 2nd Edition. Lippincott-Raven Publishers (Philadelphia).

D'Ambrosia, R.D. (ed.) (1986). *Musculoskeletal Disorders,* 2nd Edition. Lippincott (Philadelphia).

Davidoff, G.; Thomas, P.; Johnson, M.; Berent, S.; Dijkers, M.; Doljanac, R. (1988). "The Spectrum of Closed Head Injury in Acute Traumatic Spinal Cord Injury—Incidence and Risk Factors," *Arch. Phys. Med. Rehab.*

Denis, F. (1983). "Three-Column Spine and Its Significance in the Classification of Acute Thoracolumbar Spinal Injuries," *Spine* 8(8):817–831.

Duckworth, T. (1984). Lecture Notes on Orthopaedics and Fractures. Blackwell (Oxford).

Effendi, B.; Roy, D.; Cornish, B.; et al. (1981). "Fractures of the Ring of the Axis: Classification Based on Analysis of 131 Cases," *J. Bone Joint Surg.* 63B:319.

England, M.A. *Colour Atlas of the Brain and Spinal Cord.* Harcourt Health Sciences, 1991.

Galli, R.L.; Spaite, D.W.; Simon, R.R. (1989). *Emergency Orthopedics: The Spine.* Appleton & Lange (Norwalk, CT).

Gilman, S.; Winans, S.S. (1982). *Manter and Gatz's Essentials of Clinical Neuroanatomy and Neurophysiology,* 6th Edition. F.A. Davis (Philadelphia).

Greenspan, A. (1997). *Orthopedic Radiology—A Practical Approach,* 2nd Edition. Lippincott-Raven (Philadelphia).

Guyton, A.C. (1987). *Human Physiology and Mechanisms of Disease,* 4th Edition. Saunders (Philadelphia).

Hall, A.J.; Wagle, V.G.; Raycroft, J.; et al. (1993). "Magnetic Resonance Imaging in Cervical Spine Trauma," *J. Trauma* 34(1):21–26. Williams & Wilkins (Baltimore).

Harris, J.; Harris, W.; Novelline, R. (1993). *Radiology of Emergency Medicine*, 3rd Edition. Williams & Wilkins (Baltimore).

Harris, J.; Mirvis, S. (1996). *Radiology of Acute Cervical Spine Trauma*, 3rd Edition. Williams & Wilkins (Baltimore).

Helms, C. (1989). *Fundamentals of Skeletal Radiology*. Saunders (Philadelphia).

Hendee, W.R.; Ritenour, R. (1992). *Medical Imaging Physics*, 3rd Edition. Mosby Year Book (St. Louis).

Hockberger, R.; Doris, R. (1988). "Spinal Injury," in Rosen, P.; Baker, F.; Barkin, R.; et al., *Emergency Medicine: Concepts and Clinical Practice*. Mosby (St. Louis), 431–472.

Holdsworth, H. (1963). "Fractures, Dislocations and Fracture-Dislocations of Spine," *J. Bone Joint Surg.* 45B:6.

Holdsworth, H. (1970). "Fractures, Dislocations and Fracture-Dislocations of Spine," *J. Bone Joint Surg.* 52A:1534.

Hoppenfeld, S. (1977). *Orthopaedic Neurology*. Lippincott (Philadelphia).

Huebner, J. (1994). Personal communication.

Huelke, D.F. (1979). "Anatomy of the Human Cervical Spine and Associated Structures," Paper No. 790130, Society of Automotive Engineers (Warrendale, PA).

Hunt, T.K.; Goodson, W.H. (1988). "Wound Healing," Chap. 8 in Way, L.W. (ed.), *Current Surgical Diagnosis and Treatment*. Appleton & Lange (Norwalk, CT).

Hurst, J.M. (1987). *Common Problems in Trauma.* Year Book Medical Publishers (Chicago).

Jefferson, G. (1920). "Fracture of the Atlas Vertebra, Report of Four Cases and a Review of Those Previously Recorded," *Br. J. Surg.* 7:407.

Jeffreys, E. (1993). *Disorders of the Cervical Spine,* 2nd Edition. Butterworth-Heinemann Ltd. (Oxford).

Jofe, M.; White, A.; Panjabi, M. (1989). "Clinically Relevant Kinematics of Cervical Spine," in Sherk, H.H. (ed.), *The Cervical Spine,* 2nd Edition. Cervical Spine Research Society, Lippincott (Philadelphia), 57–69.

Levine, A.M.; Eismont, F.J.; Garfin, S.R.; Zigler, J.E. (1998). *Spine Trauma.* W.B. Saunders Company (Philadelphia).

Levy, R.C.; Hawkins, H.; Barsan, W.G. (1986). *Radiology in Emergency Medicine.* Mosby (St. Louis).

Mahoney, B. (1988). "Cervical Injuries," in Krome, R.; Ruiz, E., *Emergency Medicine.* McGraw-Hill (New York).

Martin, J.H. (1989). *Neuroanatomy: Text and Atlas.* Elsevier (New York).

McElhaney, J.H.; Paver, J.G.; McCrackin, H.J.; Maxwell, G.M. (1983). "Cervical Spine Compression Responses," 27th Stapp Car Crash Conference, Paper No. 831615. Society of Automotive Engineers (Warrendale, PA), 163–177.

Mirvis, S.E.; Young, J.W.R. (eds.) (1992). *Imaging in Trauma and Critical Care.* Williams & Wilkins (Baltimore).

Moore, K.L.(1985). *Clinically Oriented Anatomy,* 2nd Edition. Williams & Wilkins (Baltimore).

Myers, B.S.; McElhaney, J.H.; Richardson, W.J.; et al. (1991). "Influence of End Condition on Human Cervical Spine Injury Mechanism," 35th Stapp Car Crash Conference, Paper No. 912915. Society of Automotive Engineers (Warrendale, PA), 391–399.

Nahum, A.M.; Melvin, J.W. (eds.) (1993). *Accidental Injury: Biomechanics and Prevention.* Springer-Verlag (New York).

Netter, F.H. (1972). *The Ciba Collection of Medical Illustrations*, Vol. 1. The Ciba Collection (Summit, NJ).

Nicoll, E.A. (1949). "Fractures of the Dorso-Lumbar Spine," *J. Bone Joint Surg.* 31B(3):376–394.

Nightingale, R.W.; McElhaney, J.H.; Richardson, W.J.; et al. (1996). "Experimental Cervical Spine Injury: Relating Head Motion, Injury Classification, and Injury Mechanism," *J. Bone Joint Surg.* 78-A(3):312–421.

Nolph, M.B.; Richardson, J.D. (1987). "Cervical Injuries," Chap. 15 in Richardson, J.C.; Polk, H.C.; Flint, L.M., *Trauma: Clinical Care and Pathophysiology.* Year Book (Chicago).

Nusholtz, G.S.; Huelke, D.E.; Luz, P.; Alem, N.M.; Montavo, F. (1983). "Cervical Spine Injury Mechanisms," Proc. 27th Stapp Car Crash Conference, San Diego, CA. Society of Automotive Engineers (Warrendale, PA).

Nusholtz, G.S.; Melvin, J.W.; Huelke, D.F.; Alem, N.M.; Blank, J.O. (1981). "Response of Cervical Spine to Superior-Inferior Head Impact," 25th Stapp Car Crash Conference, Paper No. 811005. Society of Automotive Engineers (Warrendale, PA), 197–237.

Orrison, W. (1989). *Introduction to Neuroimaging.* Little Brown (Boston).

Oyesiku, N.; Amacher, A. (1990). *Patient Care in Neurosurgery.* Little Brown (Boston).

Parke, W.W.; Sherk, H.H. (1989). "Normal Adult Anatomy," in Sherk, H.H. (ed.), *The Cervical Spine*, 2nd Edition. Cervical Spine Research Society, Lippincott (Philadelphia).

Pavlov, H. (1999). *Orthopaedist's Guide to Plain Film Imaging.* Thieme (New York).

Pernkopf, E. (1963). *Atlas of Topographical and Applied Human Anatomy.* W.B. Saunders (Philadelphia).

Pike, J.A. (1989). "The Quantitative Effect of Age on Injury Outcome," Proc. 12th Experimental Safety Vehicle (ESV) Conference, Gothenburg, Sweden, May 30,1989, Paper 89-1A-W-020. NHTSA (Washington DC).

Pike, J.A. (1990). *Automotive Safety: Anatomy, Injury, Testing and Regulation,* R-171. Society of Automotive Engineers (Warrendale, PA).

Pike, J.A. (2000). "Whiplash Injury and Vehicle Design Concepts," in Yoganandan, N.; Pintar, F.A. (eds.), *Frontiers in Whiplash Trauma.* IOS Press (Netherlands), 41–45.

Pintar, F.A.; Yoganandan, N.; Voo, L.; et al. (1995). "Dynamic Characteristics of Human Cervical Spine," *SAE Transactions* 104(6):3087–3094.

Resnick, D. (1988). *Diagnosis of Bone and Joint Disorders,* 2nd Edition. Saunders (Philadelphia).

Rhea, J.; van Sonnenberg, E. (1988). *Emergency Radiology.* Little Brown (Boston).

Richardson, J.C.; Polk, H.C.; Flint, L.M. (1987). *Trauma: Clinical Care and Pathophysiology.* Year Book (Chicago).

Rockwood, C.A., Jr.; Green, D.P.; Bucholz, R.W. (1991). *Rockwood and Green's Fractures in Adults,* 3rd Edition. Lippincott (Philadephia).

Roaf, R. (1960). "Study of Mechanics of Spinal Injuries," *J. Bone Joint Surg.* 42B:810.

Rosen, P.; Baker, F.; Barkin, R.; et al. (1988). *Emergency Medicine: Concepts and Clinical Practice.* Mosby (St. Louis).

Sabiston, Jr., D.C. (1987). *Sabiston's Essentials of Surgery.* W.B. Saunders (Philadelphia).

Sadler, T.W. (1985). *Langman's Medical Embryology*, 5th Edition. Williams & Wilkins (Baltimore).

SAE (1986). "Human Tolerance to Impact Conditions as Related to Motor Vehicle Design," Information Report SAE J885 July86. Society of Automotive Engineers (Warrendale, PA).

Sherk, H.H. (ed.) (1989). *The Cervical Spine* (53 contributors), 2nd Edition. The Cervical Spine Research Society, Lippincott (Philadelphia).

Sorenson, J.A.; Phelps, M.E. (1987). *Physics in Nuclear Medicine*, 2nd Edition. Saunders (Philadephia).

Squire, L.F.; Novelline, R.A. (1988). *Fundamentals of Radiology*, 4th Edition. Harvard University Press (Cambridge).

Stauffer, E.; MacMillan, M. (1991). "Fractures and Dislocations of Spine. Part I. Cervical Spine," in Rockwood, C.; Green, D.; Bucholz, R., *Fractures in Adults*. Lippincott (Philadelphia).

Steel, H. (1968). "Anatomical and Mechanical Considerations of Atlanto-Axial Articulations," *J. Bone Joint Surg.* 50:1481–1482.

Straub, W.H. (ed.) (1989). *Manual of Diagnostic Imaging*. Little Brown (Boston).

Wamil, A.W.; Wamil, B.D.; Hellerqvist, C.G. (1998). "CM101-Mediated Recovery of Walking Ability in Adult Mice Paralyzed by Spinal Cord Injury," *Proc. Natl. Acad. Sci.* 95(22):13188–93 (Washington, DC).

Wasenko, J.J.; Lanzieri, C.F. (1992). "Plain Radiographic Examination in Cervical Spine Trauma," Chap. 6 in Camins, M.B.; O'Leary, P.F. (eds.), *Disorders of the Cervical Spine*. Williams & Wilkins (Baltimore), 53–68.

White, A.A.; Panjabi, M.M. (1990). *Clinical Biomechanics of the Spine*. Lippincott (Philadelphia).

Yoganandan, N.; Haffner, M.; Maiman, D.; et al. (1990). "Epidemiology and Injury Biomechanics of Motor Vehicle Related Trauma to the Human Spine," *SAE Transactions* 98(6):1790–1807.

Yoganandan, N.; Pintar, F.A. (eds.) (2000). *Frontiers in Whiplash Trauma: Clinical and Biomechanical.* IOS (Amsterdam).

Yoganandan, N.; Sances, Jr., A.; Pintar, F.A. (1989). "Biomechanical Evaluation of Axial Compressive Responses of Human Cadaveric and Manikin Necks," *J. Biomech. Eng.* 111(3):250–255.

Young, J.W.R.; Mirvis, S.E. (1992). "Cervical Spine Trauma," Chap. 6 in Mirvis, S.E.; Young, J.W.R. (eds.), *Imaging in Trauma and Critical Care.* Williams & Wilkins (Baltimore), 291–379.

Young, P.H. (1991). *Microsurgery of the Cervical Spine.* Raven Press (New York).

Young, W.; Ransohoff, J. (1989). "Injuries to the Cervical Cord," Chap. 7 in Sherk, H.H. (ed.), *The Cervical Spine,* 2nd Edition. The Cervical Spine Research Society, Lippincott (Philadelphia), 464–495.

Zohn, D.A. (1988). *Musculoskeletal Pain,* 2nd Edition. Little Brown (Boston), 261 pp.

Index

An abbreviation is used after the page number to indicate a footnote (*n*).

About the Author

Jeffrey A. Pike is Senior Technical Specialist, Ford Motor Company, Environmental & Safety Engineering, and Adjunct Professor, Biomedical Engineering, Wayne State University. He has 25 years of professional experience in biomechanics, human factors, human tolerance, occupant protection, testing and regulatory requirements, and the special needs of the older driver.

Mr. Pike's professional activities include: active membership in the American Association of Clinical Anatomists; the Association for the Advancement of Automotive Medicine; the International Conference on Alcohol, Drugs, and

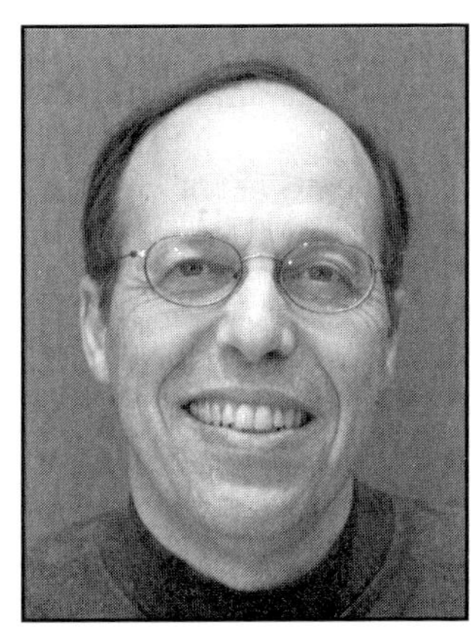

(Photo by Adam Whiteman)

Traffic Safety; and the Society of Automotive Engineers (SAE). Currently, he chairs committees for the SAE and the National Academy of Science/ Transportation Research Board and is a reviewer for U.S. Centers for Disease Control Injury Reduction Research Grant applications.

Mr. Pike has organized SAE technical conferences on various aspects of vehicular safety, as well as technical sessions at various government and industry forums, including two White House Conferences. He has served on the CDC Panel for Motor Vehicle Injury Prevention and as a consultant to the Harvard Medical School Department of Geriatrics Older Driver Program.

Mr. Pike's presentations on various aspects of automotive safety have included principal lecturer and course director for more than 50 SAE seminars and guest lectures at several schools, including the University of Michigan and Harvard Medical Schools. His publications include technical papers, book chapters, and a textbook titled *Automotive Safety: Anatomy, Injury, Testing and Regulation*, published by SAE in 1990, with its second printing in 1997. Mr. Pike's educational background includes studies at the Polytechnic Institute of New York, New York University, and the University of Michigan.